Functional Exercise Prescription

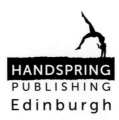

HANDSPRING
PUBLISHING
Edinburgh

Functional
Exercise
Prescription

Supporting rehabilitation in movement and sport

Eyal Lederman

Forewords Robert Schleip   Wilbour E Kelsick

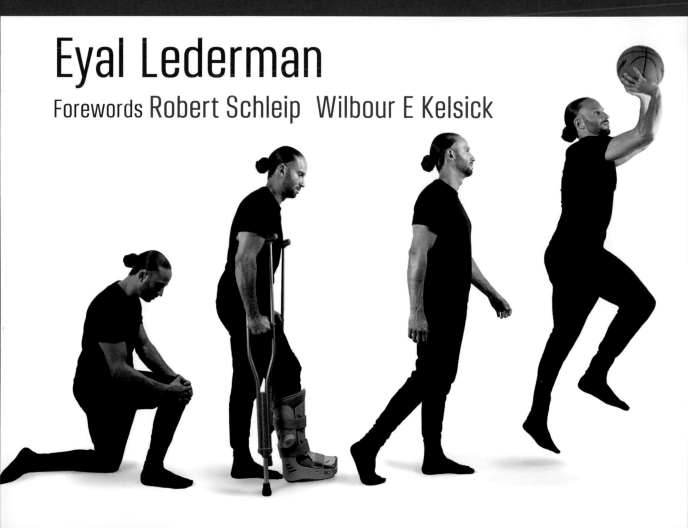

HANDSPRING PUBLISHING LIMITED
The Old Manse, Fountainhall,
Pencaitland, East Lothian
EH34 5EY, United Kingdom
Tel: +44 1875 341 859
Website: www.handspringpublishing.com

First published 2022 in the United Kingdom by Handspring Publishing

ISBN 978-1-912085-48-4
ISBN (Kindle eBook) 978-1-912085-49-1

British Library Cataloguing in Publication Data
A catalogue record for this book is available from the British Library

Library of Congress Cataloguing in Publication Data
A catalog record for this book is available from the Library of Congress

Notice
Neither the Publisher nor the Author assumes any responsibility for any loss or injury and/or damage to persons or property arising out of or relating to any use of the material contained in this book. It is the responsibility of the treating practitioner, relying on independent expertise and knowledge of the patient, to determine the best treatment and method of application for the patient.
All reasonable efforts have been made to obtain copyright clearance for illustrations in the book for which the authors or publishers do not own the rights. If you believe that one of your illustrations has been used without such clearance please contact the publishers and we will ensure that appropriate credit is given in the next reprint.

Commissioning Editor Mary Law
Project Manager Morven Dean
Copy Editor Wendy Lee
Cover, design direction and illustration Bruce Hogarth
Photography Guy Lederman
Indexer Aptara, India
Typesetter DSM, India
Printer Finidr, Czech Republic
Book set in Minion Pro Regular 12/13.5pt

The
Publisher's
policy is to use
paper manufactured
from sustainable forests

CONTENTS

ABOUT THE AUTHOR

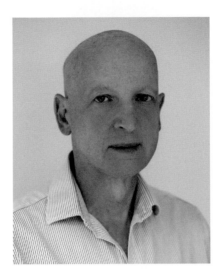

Eyal Lederman graduated from the British School of Osteopathy in 1986. Since then, he has been practicing as an osteopath in London. He completed his PhD in physiotherapy at King's College, London, where he researched the neurophysiology of manual therapy. He has also researched and developed Harmonic Technique, Functional Neuromuscular Rehabilitation, Functional Stretching, and a new clinical model in osteopathy and physical therapy called Process Approach.

Eyal is currently an Honorary Associate Professor at the Institute of Orthopaedics and Musculoskeletal Health, University College London, where he is involved in researching the clinical application of functional stretching and movement rehabilitation.

In addition to his clinical work and his research interests, Professor Lederman is the director of CPDO, a UK-based center providing continuing professional development for manual and physical therapists. Several of the manual and physical therapy approaches he developed are now taught as part of undergraduate and postgraduate training, both in the UK and elsewhere. He has published articles in the area of manual and physical therapy and is the author of the books: *Harmonic Technique; Fundamentals of Manual Therapy; The Science and Practice of Manual Therapy; Neuromuscular Rehabilitation in Manual and Physical Therapy;* and *Therapeutic Stretching: Towards a Functional Approach.* He has also contributed chapters to several other books in the fields of osteopathy and physical therapies.

DEDICATION

To Tsafi and the kids

FOREWORD BY ROBERT SCHLEIP

Beware dear reader! You are entering dangerous territory! If you are searching for orientation in the complex world of manual and movement therapies, and are hoping to find some easy guidelines that will reassure you in your beliefs then please think twice before reading further.

Let me tell you how I first got to know about the author, Dr Eyal Lederman, and how torn I was then between hating and admiring him. This was about 20 years ago, and long before I changed from being a bodywork practitioner towards becoming a fascia researcher. At that time, I earned my living as a teacher and practitioner of the Rolfing method of Structural Integration, a method of deep tissue manipulation mixed with postural education. I had attracted some respect within the Rolfing faculty and membership with a novel concept explaining how this deep tissue mobilization method might work. Contrary to the prevailing model at that time, which assumed that the manual pressure of the practitioner would be sufficient to induce a long-lasting gel-to-sol transition of the ground substance of fascial tissues, I had started to propose that the main tissue relaxation effect would more likely be due to a stimulation of Golgi tendon receptors. Stimulation of these receptors would elicit a relaxation of specific muscle fibers which then influences the resting stiffness of that same tendinous tissue. As I had some nice plausible arguments as well as anecdotal success stories at hand, I had become quite convinced and attached to that new concept and had started to teach it in my classes and beyond. But then one day, by reading an earlier book by Eyal Lederman[1], I came across a passage in which he presented clear evidence that the Golgi tendon organs do not receive sufficient stretch stimulation if the muscle fibers which are mechanically connected with them are in a relaxed condition. This is because the tendon is arranged in series with those muscle fibers. In such a dual tissue arrangement, the softer component takes over most of the overall stretch elongation while the stiffer element stays more or less the same. Unfortunately for me, Dr Lederman substantiated that analysis not only with plausible arguments but also with evidenced-based scientific references. Based on these few pages by the author, I decided to withdraw my wonderful explanatory concept, and return to the previous and less comfortable "we do not know" attitude as a humble practitioner.

Several years later, Dr Lederman stirred up a lot of heated debates when he publicly critiqued the fashionable core stability concept as "a myth".[2] That concept, which allocated a much higher importance to specific core muscles (in contrast to more superficial muscles in the same region) had become almost like a new religion for many Pilates teachers, yoga instructors and other health professionals. Not surprisingly many of these responded with less than loving feelings towards the severe arguments against their sacred beliefs. Although I had not met Dr Lederman in person at that time, I started to envision him as somebody who took a personal pleasure in being destructive and making other people angry. This impression was strengthened when he subsequently published a much discussed article on *"The fall of the postural–structural–biomechanical model in manual and physical therapies".*[3] Here too he seemed to take great pleasure in questioning – and deconstructing – many of the prevailing concepts about good posture and proper biomechanics and their importance for overall health. And again, the arguments he presented were well-formulated, well-referenced, and described in a similar manner to what you will read in this book – that is, with a very convincing and clear style of presentation.

What a surprise it was then, when I eventually met in person this man whom I had envisioned as the ultimate destroyer or as a "living knife"! I met a very charming and humble man, who was able to listen, and who treated other authors and practitioners with great respect. He enjoyed thinking deeply about almost everything, particularly about our most common assumptions. And he was also taking great diligence in developing new treatment concepts, which he had not yet published at that time.

As you read further into this book you should be willing to re-examine some of your sacred therapeutic assumptions. But more than that, you will be rewarded by novel concepts and suggestions on improving musculoskeletal health that demonstrate the opposite of a destructive attitude, by suggesting new and easy to understand concepts on health and pathology, that can be translated into daily practical applications. These include a novel focus on functional movement applications, which are particularly tailored for the individual. In addition, the book introduces a process-oriented approach, that focuses on different aspects of recovery. Rather than a sharp destructive knife, this book feels to me like the careful architectural construction of a novel foundation for future manual and movement therapy developments.

What I like the most are the author's explicit and excellent suggestions for applying the suggested principles to activities of daily living. Whether walking, standing, climbing stairs, and so forth, you will be able to practice the new functional and process-oriented principles with great pleasure in your daily life. Yes, this man is dangerous. But with this impressive book, the author provides one of the most constructive and valuable contributions towards the field of manual and movement therapies that I have known so far.

Robert Schleip
Munich, Germany
November 2021

References

1. Lederman E. *The Science and Practice of Manual Therapy*. Edinburgh: Elsevier Health Sciences; 2005.

2. Lederman E. The myth of core stability. J Bodyw Mov Ther. 2010;14:84–98.

3. Lederman E. The fall of the postural-structural-biomechanical model in manual and physical therapies: exemplified by lower back pain. J Bodyw Mov Ther. 2011;15:131-8.

It is an honour to be asked to write a foreword for Dr Eyal Lederman's book on one of the most challenging and rapidly changing sectors in healthcare in this century—exercise and rehabilitation. The validity of rehabilitative care has been challenged in the past, both in terms of its effectiveness and cost-efficiency. Rehabilitative care has now proven its rightful place but continues to face some scrutiny. I believe this book will help to minimize the criticism of rehabilitation and exercise within the healthcare field, moving it towards acceptance and validation.

In the present-day field of biological science, both the concept and the interpretation of human anatomical structure are rapidly changing. Standard traditional anatomy studies are being replaced with a more functional approach where the concepts of interrelationships between the myofascial architecture network and other body systems are highlighted or the focus. Human anatomy is no longer viewed as a static structure but rather from an integrative, functional perspective. Clinical scientists now widely accept the fact that movement is the essence of life and without it, life, in its true sense, is less than optimal, creating an environment for dysfunction and disease. Recent discoveries in the science of fascia and biotensegrity are providing more accurate interpretations of human movement and overall whole-body integrated function. Bluntly said, standard topographical anatomy is now less appealing than before, and integrated functional 3D anatomy is the new kid on the block.

This 21st century interpretation of anatomy makes it clear that movement in biological systems is not fragmented into separate compartments but functions as an integrated whole. The author highlights the concept of adaptive wholeness and its profound importance for designing personalized and condition-specific programs. He further emphasizes that adaptive changes are multidimensional in their effects on tissue, at both neurological and psychological levels; supporting integrative wholeness and not a fragmented body system. Viewing anatomy through this 21st century lens thus enables the incorporation of the interrelationship between the body's internal and external myofascial architectures and is the fundamental base on which this fascinating book is built.

In the last three decades, medical rehabilitative science has been under constant pressure to demonstrate its effectiveness within the overall healthcare paradigm. The newest concept in musculoskeletal (MSK) rehabilitation medicine is the emphasis on functional restoration rather than mere symptomatic resolution or relief. Achieving full range of motion or strength is no longer the optimal goal of treatment. However, the term "functional" is elusive in present-day rehabilitation processes if it is not structured around the need to know **why** we rehabilitate, **what** parameters we are rehabilitating, and **how** we go about rehabilitation. Unfortunately, until the why and the what are managed appropriately, the how will always be inefficient and inconsistent at all levels. This is a theme which is strongly emphasized in this book.

The main purpose of functional exercise is to "bridge the gap" between rehabilitation and a return to the same or similar levels of movement and, with the capacity to function and perform the same activities with the same skill and enjoyment as before the onset of injury or dysfunction. Eyal Lederman's classification of principles of management into functional and process approaches targeting recovery is a powerful and effective strategy. With self-healing and self-recovery as the common theme in any form of MSK dysfunction and pain recovery, such well-thought-out methodology makes logical sense as a fundamental guide for steering the complex MSK rehabilitation process. Eyal identifies three dominant processes of recovery: repair, adaptation, and alleviation of symptoms. His belief that any exercise is better than no exercise, and that the only "bad exercise" is that which fails to serve the goal of rehabilitation, is a brilliant way to encourage both therapists and patients that movement should not be feared when recovering from injury. Eyal drives home the message that even just the intent of movement is the essence of success in the rehabilitation process.

It's a great honor to have known Dr Lederman for many years and to have had the privilege to attend his workshops. His pedagogy is always clear, concise, vibrant and scientifically sound, just as it is throughout this book, in which he provides a practical and realistic approach to functional exercise as the most efficient and effective practice in rehabilitating and healing our integrated body as a whole. There are several features of this textbook that I find particularly impressive, and which brilliantly drive home the author's message:

- Chapters are organized such that the scientific background and evidence are presented first, providing a foundation for the author's thesis.
- The author's discussion of shared management highlights the concept of meaningful integration in our present healthcare system (Chapter 13).
- Chapter 14 provides detailed practical applications of the concepts and theories presented throughout the book.
- A large number of diagrams, graphs and tables that are simple to understand visually support the text.
- Comprehensive summaries at the end of each chapter serve to highlight all the important points in a concise, and easy to digest bullet-point format.

Eyal is bold in his approach but also reveals a willingness to compromise. In Chapter 7 he tackles sensitive and faddish topics about auxiliary exercises and exercise transfer, and what he refers to as its "clinical illusion". However, while Eyal believes exercise transfer has minimal benefits, he allows that any exercise movement can have some benefits, even if it's not optimal to the rehab process. This flexible approach does not alienate readers but encourages them to continue the journey into this compelling text.

Today's healthcare systems are complex, and the need for communication that facilitates an understanding of illness, therapeutic interventions, goals and outcome measures is of utmost importance. Reading this book will not only enhance your knowledge and skill about exercise prescription in rehabilitation but will also allow you to think more about why you prescribe, what you prescribe, and how you encourage your patients to adhere to their exercise programs.

I commend Dr Lederman for his effective efforts to address such a dynamic, complex and challenging topic. This piece of work is captivating and will be an effective resource and guide for accessing knowledge and fine-tuning rehabilitative skills in healthcare practitioners. I highly recommend this book to everyone with an interest in the science of exercise and rehabilitation.

Wilbour E Kelsick
Clinical Director
Maxfit Movement Institute
Port Moody, Canada

Team Practitioner
Canadian Olympic Track and Field Team

November 2021

PREFACE

My aim in writing *Functional Exercise Prescription* was to provide the reader with an understanding of the science underpinning exercise prescription and the knowledge to construct a personalized and condition-specific management for common musculoskeletal and pain conditions. There are two main themes running through the book: a *functional management* that individualizes the rehabilitation, and a *process approach* which makes it condition- and recovery-specific.

In a functional approach, all human movement is considered to be an exercise. The remedial exercises are constructed from the individual's own movement repertoire – the "life gym". Throughout life, the majority of our musculoskeletal and pain conditions recover by our daily physical activities. If these health-promoting activities are so effective, why not focus on amplifying them? It simplifies dramatically the management for the patient and supports them in attaining their own recovery goals. I came to realise early on that recovery in many musculoskeletal and pain conditions depends on three principal, whole person, processes – *repair, adaptation* and *alleviation of symptoms*. It then came to light that each of these processes requires a unique management which should be reflected in the prescribed exercise – that we need to identify the recovery process associated with the person's condition and match the exercise to support it. The outcome is a shorter and more complete recovery. This is the basis of a *process approach.*

Functional Exercise Prescription is an exercise book without "exercise." You will not find here a specific exercise to treat the ankle post-immobilization. However, you will learn how to manage this condition with the numerous activities that make up the individual's movement repertoire, and come to understand how every one of these activities, including sports, can be transformed into a remedial exercise. Yes, it is possible to manage recovery with "remedial shopping" or "remedial vacuuming", as well as "remedial tennis," "remedial soccer," yoga, or any other activity from the individual's unique functional repertoire – all activities can be amplified or attenuated according to the individual's condition.

My aim in writing *Functional Exercise Prescription* has been to shift the emphasis from traditional approaches that use exercises that are outside the individual's experience (extra-functional) towards a functional management: an approach which is more likely to support the individual's recovery needs and goals. The book is intended for use by all clinicians, including physical, manual, and sports therapists; personal trainers and team or sports coaches; and doctors and surgeons. Other health professionals, such as acupuncturists or naturopaths who would like to incorporate exercise prescription into their work, may also find this book useful. Additionally, individuals who are looking for self-care management for various musculoskeletal and pain conditions will also find it to be a useful resource. I hope it will help practitioners and their clients to construct an individualized and condition-specific management that will expedite and optimize return to functionality.

Eyal Lederman
London, UK
November 2021

There are two main themes running through the book: a *functional management* that individualizes the rehabilitation, and a *process approach* which makes it condition- and recovery-specific.

In a functional approach, all human movement is considered to be an exercise. The remedial exercises are constructed from the individual's own movement repertoire. The rehabilitation of a person following knee surgery will be constructed from their daily activities, such as standing, walking, climbing stairs, and so on. If, within their movement repertoire, they play soccer, this activity will be added to the management at some point. In this approach the patient is managed using activities that they are familiar with and which represent the ultimate goals of their rehabilitation: that is, stand, walk, play soccer. In essence, all human activities can become remedial by varying their intensity and duration. It seems that, in most conditions, maintaining daily physical activities provides the main drive for recovery. If these health-promoting activities are so effective, why not focus on amplifying them? Throughout the book these forms of exercise will be termed *functional exercise* or *functional challenges*.

A process approach is a remedial management that focuses on the processes underpinning recovery in musculoskeletal and pain conditions. Recovery in most of these conditions is associated with three dominant processes: *repair*, *adaptation*, and *alleviation of symptoms*. These recovery processes can be supported and optimized by a management that targets specific elements within the individual's environment. Exercise prescription plays an important role within the physical aspect of these environments. Each recovery process requires a specific exercise management to support it. For example,

the exercise prescribed for post-surgery rehabilitation (repair) will be very different from that for post-immobilization rehabilitation (adaptation). Some of the management elements are shared between the three recovery processes. Why and how they differ, and what is the shared management, is discussed throughout the book.

So, why is a new approach needed? Functional and process models represent a patient-centered approach where the exercises are derived from the individual's own movement repertoire and are specific to their recovery process. Exercises that are outside an individual's movement experience are termed *extra-functional* exercise/challenges/activities; sometimes, they will be referred to as *auxiliary exercise*. They are more likely to reflect the practitioner's discipline and style of practice. It is not unusual for the extra-functional exercise to be "method"-based and hijacked by fads or trends, rather than being informed by science and explored from a rational basis. Hence, currently, movement rehabilitation is dominated by exercise derived from strength and conditioning methods, Pilates, yoga, and core stability training. These approaches often promote strict exercise protocols that lack individualization or specificity to the recovery processes. These wholesale exercises are unlikely to address the person's uniqueness and their particular needs during recovery, and may therefore impede the return to functionality.

All exercises are better than no exercise. There are no "bad exercises"; there are only exercises that do not serve the goals of rehabilitation. This book is about shifting the emphasis from traditional extra-functional management towards a functional management: an approach which is more likely to support the individual's recovery needs and goals. However, there are occasions when the individual is unable to engage in functional movement. This may be due to surgical considerations (such as tendon repair), health status (autoimmunity, cancer), deficits in movement control (stroke), or environmental conditions which limit the extent of functional participation (weather conditions). Under such circumstances, extra-functional exercises play an important role in the rehabilitation program.

The book is divided into parts that reflect the functional and process approach themes. The first part (Chapters 2–3) explores functional and process approaches; the second part (Chapters 4–5) explores recovery by repair; part three (Chapters 6–9) addresses recovery by adaptation; and part four (Chapters 10–12) focuses on recovery by alleviation of symptoms. Part 5 pulls it all together: the shared management is examined in Chapter 13, while a summary, and information on how to construct functional and process approaches for common musculoskeletal and pain conditions, are provided in Chapter 14. This is supported by photographs demonstrating how the remedial exercise can be integrated into daily activities – "the life gym."

In this part of the book you will explore the basic principles of how to construct an exercise management program from the individual's own movement repertoire and how to match the management to their condition: how management can be personalized and made condition-specific.

- The principles of a functional approach (personalization of exercise)
- The principles of a process approach (how to match the exercise to the individual's recovery process)

Part 1
Principles of management

Chapter 2

Contents
A functional approach: individualizing the management

Perhaps the place to start the exploration of a functional management is to identify the goal of this rehabilitation approach. A person's functional capacity or "functionality" is seen as the ability to perform daily activities effectively, efficiently and comfortably. This capacity can be affected by various musculoskeletal and pain conditions. The aim of a functional rehabilitation is to enable the individual to regain their pre-injury capacity by using their own movement repertoire.

Imagine a session in which two patients are prescribed exercise for a similar knee injury. One patient is a keen tennis player and another a strength and conditioning enthusiast. How do we construct a functional exercise management? What would be similar and what would be different between the two presentations? How do we individualize the management? Can individualizing the exercise improve outcome? To start this exploration, we first need to look at what an exercise is.

WHAT IS AN EXERCISE?

Which of these activities would be considered an exercise: climbing a flight of stairs, walking home with shopping bags, pushing a baby carriage up a hill, repeated bending to clear clutter off the floor, cleaning the house, laying bricks, or gardening? Or would these set of activities be considered exercise: lifting weights in the gym, walking or running on a treadmill, or stretching in a yoga class?

Most people are likely to consider the first set of daily activities as undesirable daily chores. An activity would often be considered an exercise when it reaches some level of exertion and is performed in block repetitions. We also associate exercise with particular gear or sportswear,

or a dedicated space and time, such as a gym. In this mindset, exercise and sports activities are believed to confer health and fitness benefits which are not provided by daily, non-recreational activities.

From a rational point of view, all human activities provide some form of physiological, physical, and psychological challenge. What we consider to be an exercise and therefore different from daily activity is more about a mindset and context, rather than a true physiological or physical difference. From the "body's point of view," lifting a basket of washing could provide similar physical challenges to lifting a dumbbell in the gym. What forms an exercise may also depend on how incapacitated a person is. A seemingly unchallenging daily task, such as rolling out of bed, can be an exhausting exercise if the patient is very old or has been bed-ridden for several weeks. Similarly, getting in and out of a chair or walking would be a demanding challenge to a person who is recovering from lower limb surgery.

So, is there a physical activity which is not an exercise? Yes: resting or quiet sitting is considered a low metabolic activity that places minimal physical demands on the body;[1] hence, it is an activity that is unlikely to contribute to movement rehabilitation (although it is important to our well-being). However, a slow walk, which is also low on metabolic demands, could be an essential physical challenge in post-stroke or post-surgery rehabilitation. From a musculoskeletal rehabilitation perspective, it seems that all physical activities can be used to maintain, recover, or enhance performance, as well as providing wider health benefits. These considerations form the basis for broad definitions of exercise and remedial exercise:

Exercise is the behavior a person adopts in order to maintain or enhance their physical performance or health.

Remedial exercise is the behavior a person adopts in order to recover their physical performance or health.

These definitions encompass the notion that all human activity, including mundane daily tasks, can be considered remedial exercise and therefore beneficial for recovery. But is there any evidence for this?

THE BENEFITS OF THE MUNDANE

The first question that comes to mind is how individuals who do not engage in a structured recreational exercise regime maintain their physical capacity to carry out daily activities. How do we maintain our ability to climb a flight of stairs without special exercise? It seems that, by simply performing daily tasks, we attain and maintain our capacity to perform them (Fig. 2.1A&B). Walking maintains walking; getting in and out of chairs maintains this ability; bending, twisting, and reaching maintain our

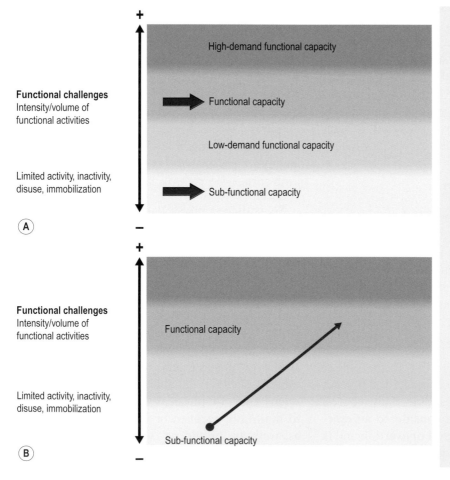

FIGURE 2.1
Functional activities maintain functional capacity. (A) In conditions such as immobilization, disuse, and neglect, functional engagement is lowered to a "sub-functional" capacity. (B) Often, movement rehabilitation revolves around recovering functional capacity from the sub-functional level. Importantly, this can be achieved simply by gradually increasing the intensity and volume of the individual's functional activities.

agility, and so on. Most of these daily tasks are usually performed within a comfort zone. Occasionally, we might experience discomfort, such as fatigue when we over-exert ourselves – say, with a long walk. On the other hand, sports-related activities are largely associated with physical exertion, discomfort, and even pain, such as when we experience "muscle burn" or become acutely and painfully out of breath. On the whole, daily tasks do not provide this exertion experience to the same extent, and hence most individuals would not consider them to be

health-enhancing activities (think vacuuming). This distinction, however, is far from the physiological reality.

It is well established that many of our daily activities provide substantial challenges which maintain our physical capacity. This is exemplified in Figure 2.2, which demonstrates the physical forces imposed on the knee by daily and recreational activities. A basic daily activity such as walking, loads the knee by 2.6 times our body weight (BW), getting up from sitting by 2.5xBW,

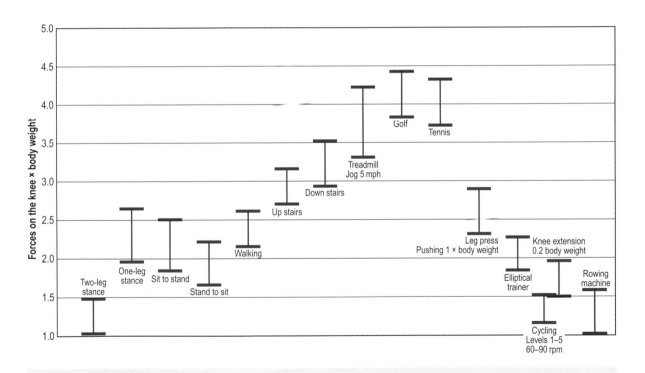

FIGURE 2.2

Forces exerted on the knee during daily and recreational activities. (Adapted from Kutzner I, Heinlein B, Graichen F, Bender A, Rohlmann A, Halder A, et al. Loading of the knee joint during activities of daily living measured in vivo in five subjects. J Biomech. 2010;43:2164–73; and D'Lima DD, Steklov N, Patil S, Colwell CW. The Mark Coventry Award: in vivo knee forces during recreation and exercise after knee arthroplasty. Clin Orthop Relat Res. 2008;466:2605–11.)

and descending stairs by 3.5xBW.[2–5] Such loading forces are also seen in other areas of the body. In the glenohumeral (GH) joint, lifting a kettle weighing 1.4 kg loads the joint by 1xBW: the equivalent of the whole of our body weight passes through that joint (Fig. 2.3). A simple activity such as combing our hair produces loads of 0.6–0.9xBW in the GH joint.[5] Similarly, in the lumbar spine, when comparing loading forces of standing to other daily activities, it was found that walking increases vertebral loading by 1.7 xBW, ascending stairs by 2.6 xBW and descending stairs by 2.2 xBW, getting out of a chair by 3.8 xBW, and turning from side-lying to a supine position, and vice versa, by 2.2xBW.[6,7] In the metacarpophalangeal joint, a simple daily task such as gripping a pen can generate dramatic loading stresses equal to forces observed in some hip activities.[8] Such loading patterns are expected in many other joints during a variety of daily tasks.

The health benefits of daily activities can be observed beyond the musculoskeletal system. This phenomenon has been shown in studies that explore the benefits of moderate-intensity activities of daily living (active transportation, occupation, or domestic duties) and recreational physical activities (sports, gym, and so on) on overall mortality and major cardiovascular disease.[9–12] In one major study with 130,000 participants, it was found that both moderate recreational and non-recreational activities are associated with a lower risk for mortality and major cardiovascular events, regardless of the type of physical activity.[10] Longer weekly exposure to moderate non-recreational activities was shown to confer cumulative cardiovascular health benefits, surpassing even those observed in moderate recreational sports activities (Fig. 2.4A&B).

The above research findings highlight the importance of daily activities in maintaining both systemic and musculoskeletal health. These benefits are seen even in individuals who are not engaged in recreational exercise or sports activities. This suggests that engaging in daily activities can provide adequate physical challenges to maintain their performance.

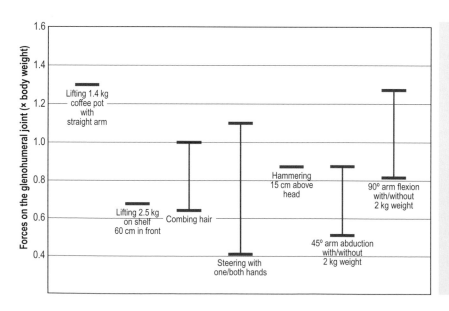

FIGURE 2.3

Forces exerted on the glenohumeral joint during daily activities. (Adapted from Bergmann G, Graichen F, Bender A, Kääb M, Rohlmann A, Westerhoff P. In vivo glenohumeral contact forces: measurements in the first patient 7 months postoperatively. J Biomech. 2007;40:2139–49.)

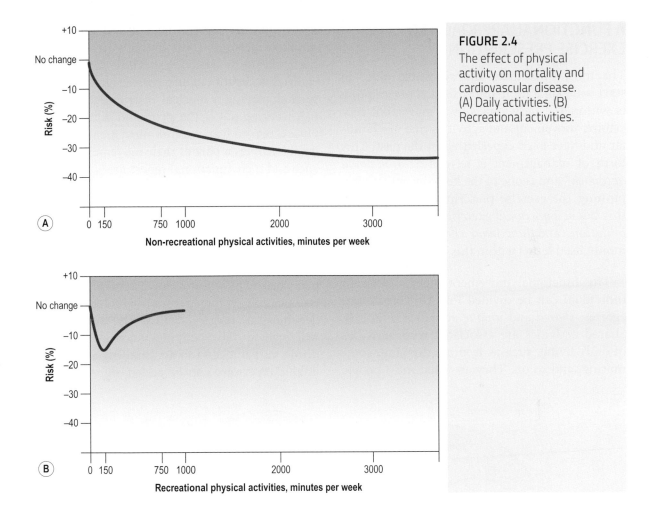

FIGURE 2.4
The effect of physical activity on mortality and cardiovascular disease. (A) Daily activities. (B) Recreational activities.

By walking we maintain our walking capacity, by daily bending, lifting, twisting, and reaching we maintain our agility and ability to perform these tasks – no other exercise is required. This phenomenon is seen throughout a person's functional repertoire. This notion provides us with a very important principle when constructing an exercise prescription program: start off the exercise management with the functional repertoire whenever possible (see exceptions below). Since functional activities maintain functionality, they also offer the elementary challenges to support

recovery. This is the essence of a functional management. It engages the person in daily activities that challenge their functional losses. The message to the patient is simple and clear – practice what you aim to recover (or, practice *only* what you aim to recover?). We can observe that most people recover from most of their injuries, most of the time, by simply engaging in the activities that have been affected by their condition. So, if daily activities can potentially be such an effective therapeutic tool, how do we choose these challenges? Where do we start?

A FUNCTIONAL APPROACH TO EXERCISE PRESCRIPTION

The most immediate and accessible place to start an exploration into exercise prescription is within the individual's own movement repertoire: movement and activities that are familiar and have been experienced in the past. This form of management is termed a *"functional approach"* and is one of the key concepts underpinning the exercise prescription described in this book. *Functional exercise*, *functional rehabilitation*, and *functional challenges* are commonly used terms within this approach.

The functional movement repertoire of an individual can be divided into two broad categories: *shared* and *unique* activities (Fig. 2.5). Shared activities are associated with activities of daily living, such as feeding, dressing, commuting, and so on. They are what most people do within their shared sociocultural realm. The unique repertoire contains activities that are particular to the individual. These include specialized occupational and recreational activities such as playing a musical instrument, gardening, working out at the gym, and doing sports. Once a person learns a new movement or activity, it becomes a part of their movement experience and their functional repertoire.

Most individuals who experience musculoskeletal and pain conditions express a wish to be able to return to their pre-injury physical ability. Hence, a functional exercise prescription aims to help the person recover their movement capacity by using their own movement repertoire whenever possible. For a person who has had a shoulder injury or surgery, the exercise prescription will include daily activities such as reaching, lifting, carrying, and so on. Challenges from the unique repertoire can be added, depending on

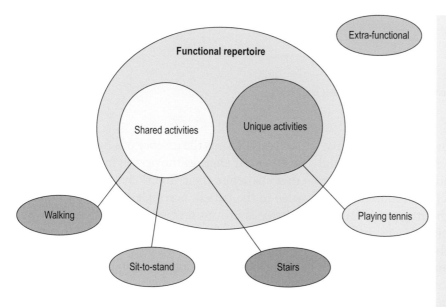

FIGURE 2.5

A person's functional repertoire represents their total movement experiences – activities which they are familiar with. It contains a range of shared and unique activities. Activities outside the individual's movement experience are extra-functional. In functional rehabilitation the remedial exercises are constructed from the person's movement repertoire.

their stage of recovery. They can be in the form of graded challenges, such as using tennis to rehabilitate a tennis player or a progressive workout with weights for the gym enthusiast. This personal repertoire is the basis for individualizing exercise prescription. Why invent something new? Use what the person has already knows and is used to.

CONSTRUCTING A FUNCTIONAL EXERCISE MANAGEMENT PROGRAM

How do we construct an exercise plan within a functional approach? Do we need to know specific exercises for certain areas of the body or particular pathologies? How do upper limb exercises differ from lower limb or trunk exercise? From where do we source the remedial exercise?

These questions can be resolved by looking at the regional functionality of an area such as the lower limbs (Fig. 2.6A–C). Within the shared repertoire, the lower extremity is used in activities such as getting up from sitting, standing, walking, climbing stairs, and so on. Hence, regardless of the underlying condition or pathology, the knee has to flex, extend, and rotate in all leg activities, in the context of what the person does with their leg within their environment: sit to stand, walk, climb stairs, and so on. Now, imagine two patients, each presenting with a different knee condition: say, post-operative cruciate and meniscus repair. Would the management differ between the two conditions? In both conditions the physiological movement ranges of the knee have to recover (flexion, extension, and rotation), but also the knee has to participate in all the functional weight-bearing activities. Hence, the exercise prescription for the two conditions would be exactly the same. This principle applies to any knee condition, regardless of the underlying pathology. A person who has had

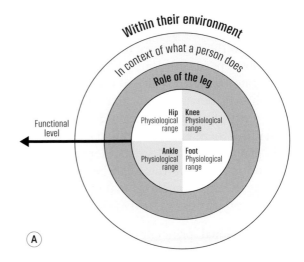

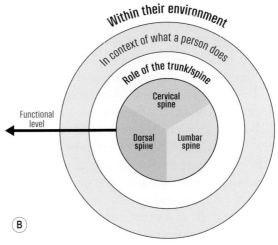

FIGURE 2.6

Context principle in constructing a functional exercise rehabilitation. (A) For the lower limb. (B) For the spine/trunk. (A and B, After Lederman E. Neuromuscular rehabilitation in manual and physical therapy. Edinburgh: Churchill Livingstone; 2010.)

acute sprain, osteoarthritis, knee replacement, or meniscal repair still has to be able to flex, extend, and rotate the knee, stand up, walk, and so on. But what about ankle rehabilitation: would it be different to the above knee management? From a functional perspective, all the lower limb joints participate in the activities of daily living. The ankle has to dorsiflex and plantar-flex within the context of what the person does with their leg within their environment: e.g., stand up, walk, play football, and so on. Hence, all lower limb joints and conditions can be managed by applying this functional regional repertoire – no need for complex or exhaustive exercise regimes.

This regional principle can be applied for managing various upper limb conditions. Within the shared functional repertoire, the upper limb is used typically for reaching, grasping, and retrieving, carrying and manipulating objects, and so on. From a functional perspective, the shoulder, elbow, wrist, and hands are all involved in this repertoire. This means that in all upper limb conditions the exercise prescription will be similar, regardless of the anatomical location, joints, tissues involved, or even the nature of the underlying pathology: e.g., a person with frozen shoulder, or subacromial decompression, or post-shoulder dislocation surgery, still has to recover daily tasks that require reaching and retrieving movements.

What about the spine – or, more correctly, the trunk? Would the prescribed exercise change if two patients presented with conditions in different locations: say, dorsal and lumbar spine? The answer to this clinical conundrum can be explored with another question: is there any human activity in which the trunk is left out? The whole of the trunk is involved in all human activities, from walking, lifting, bending, twisting, reaching, and using stairs to playing

tennis, and so on. It difficult to imagine an activity in which the trunk is not under some form of mechanical loading or in complete muscle silence (even lying down we use our trunk muscles for breathing). This means that all activities within a person's functional repertoire can be used to challenge the spine/trunk – no need for back-specific exercise. Hence, the dorsal and lumbar spine can be rehabilitated using the same daily activities. But what about a person who presents with lumbar spine discectomy and another who has had abdominal or heart surgery? Would the management of the anterior and posterior aspects of the torso be the same or different? Since the trunk, as a whole, participates in all human movements, all these activities can be part of the remedial care. This means that all functional activities can be used to manage recovery from any condition or pathology afflicting any part of the torso.

Exercise prescription for neck conditions can follow the same principles described above. Although the neck is involved in all functional tasks, it is also has the unique job of supporting the head in movements associated with tracking the senses: sight, taste, and hearing. This function can be utilized to challenge neck movements. For example, neck rotation can be challenged by simply following the gaze to the right and left while sitting or standing, or walking with the head slightly turned to the affected side. There is no physiological difference between giving a patient a neck rotation exercise or a functional task such as turning the head when parking the car.

From the above examples it can be seen that the body may be divided into four major functional regions: lower limbs, upper limbs, torso/trunk, and head and neck (Fig. 2.7). Each of these regions has a unique role within any given task. This, somewhat artificial, division

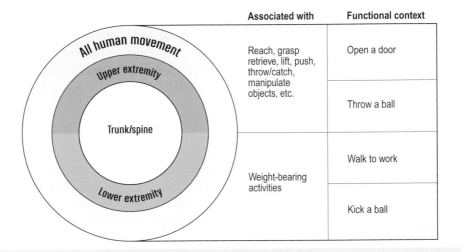

FIGURE 2.7
The whole body plays a role in the functional repertoire. However, there are functional regions that are associated with the ability to perform specific tasks: lower limbs, upper limbs, torso/trunk, and head and neck. Each of these regions has a unique role within the context of any given task. Exercise prescription is constructed from these functional roles. However, in functional rehabilitation the aim is to enable the patient to recover their capacity to perform the affected task(s), so in most exercise prescription all the regions play a part in the task: for example, a simple side-reaching exercise for the arm can be used to rehabilitate the arm, trunk, and legs.

provides a convenient clinical tool; it dramatically simplifies the planning of an exercise prescription program. The therapist is no longer required to construct a specific rehabilitation for every pathology in any of these four regions. Prescription is given according to the role that each of these regions plays within the affected tasks, as described in the above examples.

EXTRA-FUNCTIONAL MANAGEMENT

Traditional forms of exercise prescription are mostly based on strength and conditioning principles. They are often very different from the individual's functional repertoire or goals of recovery. It is not unusual for a patient recovering from leg surgery or injury to be given exercises such as seated leg bench-presses or extension exercise using resistance bands. These exercises bear no resemblance to functional human activities and are likely to be outside the individual's movement experiences. In a functional approach the term *"extra-functional"* refers to movements and activities which are unfamiliar to the individual and outside their functional repertoire.

To make a point by way of exaggeration: imagine prescribing an extra-functional exercise such as soccer to a tennis player recovering from a leg injury. This management would seem misplaced and ineffective. Similarly, it would be considered unsuitable to prescribe tennis for a runner with leg injuries or to prescribe rock climbing for a tennis player with shoulder injuries. Yet, paradoxically, it is common to see an extra-functional exercise prescription which bears no resemblance to the activities the individual aims to recover (termed *goal activity*). For example, patients with low back conditions are commonly prescribed extra-functional exercise such as core stability training on the floor or exercise ball, complex stretching, strength training with gym equipment or resistance bands, and so on. All these activities bear no resemblance to the functional repertoire of most individuals. Traditional rehabilitation literature and training practices are dominated by extra-functional management. It seems that the more outlandish the exercise is and the further it is from recognizable functional activities, the more therapeutic value is placed on it. But how useful are these extra-functional approaches for rehabilitating the functional repertoire, activities such as getting out of a chair, standing, walking, and so on? How close does the remedial exercise need to be, in order to benefit the goal activity the person aims to recover?

For close on a century, research has been exploring how similar the training and the goal activity have to be. The message so far from the sciences is very clear: there are greater benefits when the prescribed exercise closely resembles the goal activity. Even minor dissimilarities between the two can reduce the carry-over (transfer) of training gains to the goal activity. This phenomenon was observed in skill acquisition, and human and sports performance, as well as movement rehabilitation (see Chapter 7).[12] For example, in stroke rehabilitation, recent guidelines recommended that interventions should favor task-specific training.[13] Importantly, it was noted that improvements are mostly within the functions and activities a person has been trained in; essentially, we only learn or improve what we have practiced (we are unlikely to learn or improve something we have not practiced).

A similar ineffective carry-over of training gains was reported in a recent review of functional rehabilitation in the elderly.[14] It was found that the commonly prescribed resistance exercises (extra-functional) have a limited contribution to activities of daily living, whereas a functional rehabilitation was shown to be more beneficial.

There are occasions when transfer of training gains is seen between dissimilar activities; however, they tend to be rare and unpredictable.[12] Hence, a functional approach removes this uncertainty and simplifies the selection of prescribed exercises. Essentially, if the training is in the form of the goal activity, it tends to minimize the reliance on transfer. It also dramatically simplifies the management!

Benefits of functional versus extra-functional management

There are several important benefits in a functional exercise management in comparison to an extra-functional one. A functional approach uses the individual's own movement resources and therefore does not require additional learning and ongoing instruction. On the other hand, extra-functional exercises are unfamiliar to the individual. The individual has to learn a new set of activities at a time when they are least able to – often, when they are experiencing pain and loss of movement capacity. Learning requires set-aside time, intense mental focus, and physical effort. Extra-functional approaches create an unfavorable situation in which the individual is highly dependent on others for instructions and guidance, at least during the training period. We have to keep in mind that 40–80% of medical instructions are forgotten immediately after the session, and 50% remembered incorrectly; the more we pile on the information, the less is remembered.[15,16] Considering all these factors, no wonder patients often forget how to perform the exercise they have been given. So, keeping it simple and familiar is important.

A functional approach could support compliance and adherence by engaging the individual in activities that are important to them (see Chapter 13).[17–21] A keen tennis player will be happy and highly motivated to participate in a management that centers on "remedial tennis," but it may be a struggle to get them to exercise in a gym. Hence, compliance and adherence can be enhanced by selecting the movement challenges from the patient's own functional repertoire. Not sure which? Just ask the patient which activities they are keen to get back to.

Functional rehabilitation has important implications for training accessibility. In a functional approach the movement challenges are integrated into the person's daily activities and can be practiced anywhere and at any time. Movement challenges are all around, within their environment. Essentially, their life becomes their gym. The functional program seldom relies on any specialized exercise equipment or dedicated space. Everyday objects and activities can be used to challenge movement losses. Treadmill machines can be expensive while level walking is free. A functional approach is inexpensive and easy to apply, and simplifies self-care.

From a therapist's perspective, a functional approach simplifies the clinical management when faced with the myriad of extra-functional exercise possibilities. To take the leg as an example, there is no need to remember exercises specifically for the hip, knee, foot, ankle, or particular muscles in the leg. Additionally, there is rarely a need-to-know special exercise for every leg pathology. All that we need to remember is that the person has to get up from sitting, stand, walk, climb stairs (shared repertoire), and

eventually kick a soccer ball (unique repertoire), regardless of the anatomical structure or the pathology afflicting it. However, an understanding of the processes by which the individual will recover from their condition and regain their functionality is important for the management. This is the basis for the process approach discussed in the next chapter.

Functional exercise brings about whole-body adaptation that helps the recovery and supports the individual's functional capacity. Such functional adaptation does not take place in extra-functional exercises. This may account for some of the limitations of these practices for providing meaningful recovery results; see Chapters 6 and 7 for further discussion of adaptation to exercise, training specificity, and transfer of training gains.

Importance of extra-functional management

There are many occasions where an extra-functional exercise has an important role in the remedial plan, particularly in acute post-injury/surgery conditions where, initially, it is necessary to reduce the forces imposed on the damaged tissues: for example, off-weight-bearing exercise after lower limb tendon surgery. However, once weight-bearing activities are considered safe, the management should move from extra-functional to functional exercise. In principle, if the patient is able to walk into the clinic there is no point in introducing off-weight-bearing movement challenges such as seated bench presses, and so on. Once a person is functional, there is no need to regress the management to the extra-functional.

Additionally, there are circumstances in which the individual is unable to perform functional activities due to health limitations or environmental circumstances, such as stroke or limited

a vertebral body replacement during locomotion measured in vivo. Gait Posture. 2014;39:750–5.

8. Butz KD, Merrell G, Nauman EA. A three-dimensional finite element analysis of finger joint stresses in the MCP joint while performing common tasks. Hand (N Y). 2012;7:341–5.

9. Ekblom-Bak E, Ekblom B, Vikström M, de Faire U, Hellénius ML. The importance of non-exercise physical activity for cardiovascular health and longevity. Br J Sports Med. 2014;48:233–8.

10. Lear SA, Hu W, Rangarajan S, Gasevic D, Leong D, Iqbal R, et al. The effect of physical activity on mortality and cardiovascular disease in 130 000 people from 17 high-income, middle-income, and low-income countries: the PURE study. Lancet 2017;390:2643–54.

11. Soares-Miranda L, Siscovick DS, Psaty BM, Longstreth WT, Mozaffarian D. Physical activity and risk of coronary heart disease and stroke in older adults: the Cardiovascular Health Study. Circulation 2016;133:147–55.

12. Schmidt RA, Lee TD. Motor control and learning. 4th ed. Stanningley, UK: Human Kinetics; 2005.

13. Veerbeek JM, van Wegen E, van Peppen R, van der Wees PJ, Hendriks E, Rietberg M, et al. What is the evidence for physical therapy poststroke? A systematic review and meta-analysis. PLoS One. 2014;9:e87987.

14. Liu C, Shiroy DM, Jones LY, Clark DO. Systematic review of functional training on muscle strength, physical functioning, and activities of daily living in older adults. Eur Rev Aging Phys Act. 2014;11:144.

15. Kessels RP. Patients' memory for medical information. J R Soc Med. 2003;96:219–22.

16. Anderson JL, Dodman S, Kopelman M, Fleming A. Patient information recall in a rheumatology clinic. Rheumatol Rehabil. 1979;18:18–22.

17. Schneider RC, Aiken FA. Effects of selected personal environmental, and activity characteristics on exercise adherence. Available from: http://www.naturalspublishing.com/files/published/p33k3844t7dw35.pdf.

18. Chan DK, Lonsdale C, Ho PY, Yung PS, Chan KM. Patient motivation and adherence to post-surgery rehabilitation exercise recommendations: the influence of physiotherapists' autonomy–supportive behaviors. Arch Phys Med Rehabil. 2009;90:1977–82.

19. Minor MA, Brown JD. Exercise maintenance of persons with arthritis after participation in a class experience. Health Educ Behav. 1993;20:83–95.

20. Jolly K, Taylor R, Lip GYh, Greenfield S, Raftery J, Mant J, et al. The Birmingham Rehabilitation Uptake Maximisation Study (BRUM). Home-based compared with hospital-based cardiac rehabilitation in a multi-ethnic population: cost-effectiveness and patient adherence. Health Technol Assess. 2007;11:1–118.

21. Schwarzer R, Luszczynska A, Ziegelmann JP, Scholz U, Lippke S. Social-cognitive predictors of physical exercise adherence: three longitudinal studies in rehabilitation. Health Psychol. 2008;27:S54–S63.

22. World Health Organization. Global strategy on diet, physical activity and health. Physical inactivity: a global public health problem; 2019. Available from: https://www.who.int/dietphysicalactivity/factsheet_inactivity/en/.

23. Lederman E. Neuromuscular rehabilitation in manual and physical therapy. Edinburgh: Churchill Livingstone; 2010, p. 178.

24. Lederman E. The fall of the postural-structural-biomechanical model in manual and physical therapies: exemplified by lower back pain. J Bodyw Mov Ther. 2011;15:131–8.

Chapter 3

Contents

A process approach: constructing a condition-specific management program

Imagine these three common clinical scenarios: a patient who has just had knee joint surgery; another who has had 8 weeks of knee immobilization; and a third who has chronic knee pain associated with moderate arthritis – three different conditions in the same anatomical location. How would the exercise prescription differ between them? Are there management elements which are shared or specific to all these different conditions? What guides us in selecting suitable exercise for the individual's condition?

There is a theme connecting the recovery in all musculoskeletal and pain conditions – the awe-inspiring capacity of the body/person to initiate self-healing and self-recovery processes. The success of any physical therapy management, including exercise prescription, is highly dependent on these recovery processes. These recovery processes are the therapeutic target of a process-focused rehabilitation. Hence, the rehabilitation of a person who has sprained their ankle is primarily directed at supporting the processes that will lead to their recovery: repair.

In a process-led management, the aim is to identify condition-related recovery processes and create with the patient environments that support them. These environments are multi-dimensional, containing physical, behavioral, psychological, and social components. Physical activities and exercise are seen as part of this recovery environment.

THE THREE RECOVERY PROCESSES

A process approach takes the view that a person can recover from their musculoskeletal and pain conditions by three primary processes, namely: *repair*, *adaptation*, and *alleviation of symptoms* (Fig. 3.1).[1] If a person sprains their knee, say, or has surgery, they will expect to recover

their functionality through the process of tissue repair.[2–5] On the other hand, if a person is immobilized following a knee fracture, it will result in multisystem adaptive changes, affecting all musculoskeletal tissues, neuromuscular control, and vascular and lymphatic systems.[6–9] The subsequent functional recovery after removal of the cast will also be dependent on adaptive processes affecting all these tissues and systems.[6,10–12]

In the next example, a person with mild osteoarthritis of the knee has been experiencing chronic pain for several months. Within a few weeks of treatment there is a dramatic improvement in their condition. Supposing the knee was X-rayed before the onset of treatment and again, several weeks later, when the person is pain-free. Would we see a "before" and "after" difference in the imaging? It is very likely that the X-ray findings will remain unchanged: the underlying joint pathology will still be evident. This phenomenon is observed in many chronic musculoskeletal conditions, such as long-term low back pain and tendinopathies.[13–18] It seems that functional capacity can recover, despite permanent tissue pathology, e.g., the presence of osteoarthritic changes. So, the question is, by which process has the person recovered their functionality in this scenario? We can eliminate repair and tissue adaptation. It is well established that tissue repair, particularly the painful inflammatory phase, lasts from a few days to about 2 weeks (excluding autoimmune conditions and so on). This means that in chronic pain conditions that persist for several months or years, the mechanism maintaining the pain experience is unlikely to be related to repair processes, or that recovery from chronic pain is unlikely to be through resolution of repair (see Chapter 10). It is also improbable that recovery happens through adaptive tissue changes. Such pathological structural

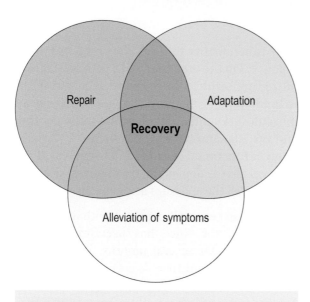

FIGURE 3.1
Functional recovery from musculoskeletal and pain conditions is brought about by three primary processes, namely: *repair, adaptation,* and *alleviation of symptoms.*

changes in joint surfaces or spine (osteoarthritis, disk degeneration and so on) are unlikely to regenerate and normalize in any meaningful way to account for a functional recovery. So, is there another option for functional recovery in the presence of unshakeable pathology?

This leaves the possibility that recovery can take place solely through alleviation or modulation of symptoms: a recovery process different from tissue repair or adaptation.[19–21] Imagine this analogy: a person with a headache or back pain takes a painkiller (or placebo). For a period of time, they will experience an improvement in their condition and, being pain-free, resume their daily activities. Yet the underlying cause of their painful condition is still there; it is just that they are no longer aware of it. From the individual's

point of view, at that point in time they have been "cured" of their condition. So, functional improvement can take place via symptomatic change, even without a change in the degree or nature of the underlying pathology, i.e., a symptomatic recovery rather than a "cure."

Most musculoskeletal and pain conditions improve through one or a combination of the three recovery processes (Fig. 3.2A; Table 3.1). Any condition where there is recent traumatic tissue damage is principally associated with recovery by repair.[22] Recovery by repair includes conditions such as acute spinal and disk injuries, nerve root irritation, joint/capsular–ligamentous sprains or strains, muscle tears, and so on. This form of recovery will be further discussed in Chapter 4.

Recovery by adaptation is largely associated with persistent, long-term conditions and the latter remodeling phase of repair. Adaptation processes underlie recovery in conditions such as post-immobilization, long-term contractures after injury and surgery, and the stiff phase of frozen shoulder.[23–26] This form of recovery is seen in central nervous system damage, such as stroke and traumatic head injuries. Central nervous system plasticity, motor learning, and habitual or behavioral changes are also associated with adaptive processes. Hence, long-term transformation of posture, task learning, and enhancing skill and sports performance are all dependent on the body's adaptive capacity. Recovery by adaptation is further discussed in Chapter 6.

Symptomatic related recovery plays an important role in recuperation from most chronic conditions, such as low back and neck pain,[13,15–18] symptomatic relief in osteoarthritis,[27–29] improvements in painful tendinopathies,[30–32] and

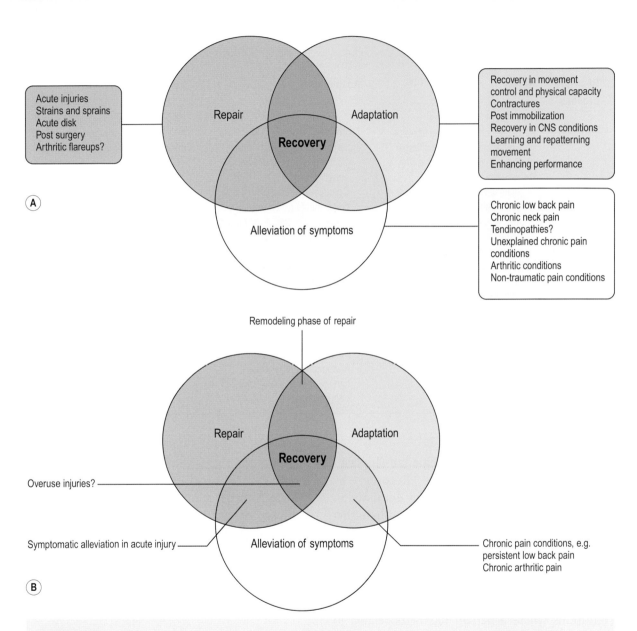

Acute injuries
Strains and sprains
Acute disk
Post surgery
Arthritic flareups?

Repair

Adaptation

Recovery

Recovery in movement
control and physical capacity
Contractures
Post immobilization
Recovery in CNS conditions
Learning and repatterning
movement
Enhancing performance

Alleviation of symptoms

Chronic low back pain
Chronic neck pain
Tendinopathies?
Unexplained chronic pain
conditions
Arthritic conditions
Non-traumatic pain conditions

Ⓐ

Remodeling phase of repair

Repair

Adaptation

Recovery

Overuse injuries?

Symptomatic alleviation in acute injury

Alleviation of symptoms

Chronic pain conditions, e.g.
persistent low back pain
Chronic arthritic pain

Ⓑ

FIGURE 3.2
Conditions and their related recovery processes. (A) Recovery processes associated with common musculoskeletal and pain conditions. (B) Conditions associated with overlapping recovery processes.

Recovery process	Repair	Adaptation	Symptomatic modulation
Condition	All acute conditions and flareups within the time frame of inflammation, proliferation, and early remodeling, e.g.: All tissue damage Acute pain (with/without injury) Joint and muscle sprains Acute low back and neck pain, including disk-related conditions Post-surgery Blunt trauma Painful phase of frozen shoulder Acute tendinopathies Acute flareups in persistent pain conditions, e.g. low back and arthritis Overuse injuries?	All conditions affecting functional capacity and performance, e.g.: Conditions affecting task performance Conditions affecting task components (force, endurance, speed and range of movement, balance and coordination) Post-immobilization, detraining Range of movement loss, e.g. stiff phase of frozen shoulder Induction of structural/biomechanical change Chronic tendinopathies? Central nervous system damage Postural and movement re-education/rehabilitation enhance/recover task performance	All persistent symptoms beyond the expected repair duration, e.g.: All persistent, pain, discomfort and stiffness experiences Chronic low back and neck pain Chronic arthritic pain Chronic tendinopathies? Overuse injuries?

Table 3.1 Associated recovery processes in common musculoskeletal and pain conditions

other unexplained local and regional whiplash-associated pain conditions.[33,34] Recovery by modulation of symptoms is further discussed in Chapters 10 and 11. It should be noted here that return to functionality can take place, even in the absence of symptomatic improvements. This can occur through psychological processes where there is a shift in the person's attitude or relationship to their pain. This is seen in chronic pain conditions where a person has fears related to pain and movement. By overcoming these anxieties, through activities such as exercise, they may re-engage in functional activities, although their pain levels may remain unchanged.

Functional recovery through symptomatic modulation is not limited to pain experience. It includes other symptoms of "dis-ease," such as stiffness, paresthesia, and affective experiences such as anxiety and depression. However, for the purpose of finishing this book, the focus will be on pain and stiffness experiences.

OVERLAPPING PROCESSES

Recuperation in a variety of conditions is often associated with a combination of recovery processes. This is depicted by the overlap areas of the Venn diagram in Figure 3.2B. In clinical reality, several of these processes may overlap in any given condition, often with one of the three processes being more dominant.

The overlap between repair and adaptation represents the recovery associated with remodeling of tissues after injury. Initially, repair is dominated by an inflammatory phase that, in time, shifts towards proliferation and a latter remodeling process.[22] The remodeling phase, in particular, is largely adaptive in nature and serves to restore the tissues' biomechanical and physiological properties. During this phase, musculoskeletal tissues continually remodel in response to the individual's physical interaction with their environment.[35–43]

The overlap between repair and modulation of symptoms is associated with alleviation of pain and stiffness in acute conditions. This recovery is partly the resolution of inflammation and a gradual attenuation of nociceptive excitation at the site of damage. Some of the symptomatic improvements are associated with diminishing central and peripheral sensitization (see Chapter 10).[21] This area of overlap also represents recovery in motor or sensory symptoms arising from peripheral neuropathies. Symptomatic recovery in these conditions is dependent on successful resolution of repair in the affected nerve or surrounding tissues or structures, such as nerve root compression in disk injuries.

The overlap between adaptation and modulation of symptoms represents recovery in most chronic musculoskeletal and pain conditions. Chronic pain conditions are often associated with central sensitization – a process related to neuroplasticity and adaptation (see Chapter 10).[21] This form of recovery process is seen in conditions such as chronic low back and neck pain, persistent post-operative pain, and osteoarthritis. Recovery in these conditions is likely to be due to long-term desensitization – an adaptive central nervous system process associated with neuroplasticity.[21]

MULTIDIMENSIONAL RECOVERY ENVIRONMENT

Imagine an individual who has had a plaster cast removed after ankle fracture. Their functional recovery will be highly dependent on weight-bearing activities such as walking and climbing stairs. This behavior, in turn, depends on cognitive and psychological factors, motivation, needs, and functional goals: "get back to work, be able to play tennis again," and so on. But this recovery behavior is also dependent on multiple environmental factors, which include social (going out with friends), occupational (walk to work), and recreational opportunities (cycling, running). A process approach aims to create, with the patient, environments in which their recovery processes can be supported and optimized (Fig. 3.3). It contains management that is unique to each recovery process, as well as management that is shared by all three processes (see Chapter 13; Fig. 3.4). The recovery environments contain physical, behavioral, psychological–cognitive, and social–cultural dimensions. Exercise and activities that challenge the individual's movement deficits form an important part of the physical aspect of this environment. These management considerations are discussed in the following chapter.

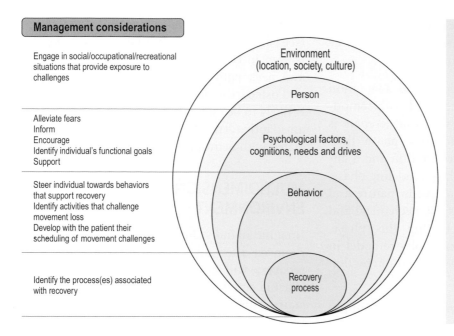

Management considerations

Engage in social/occupational/recreational situations that provide exposure to challenges

Alleviate fears
Inform
Encourage
Identify individual's functional goals
Support

Steer individual towards behaviors that support recovery
Identify activities that challenge movement loss
Develop with the patient their scheduling of movement challenges

Identify the process(es) associated with recovery

Environment
(location, society, culture)

Person

Psychological factors, cognitions, needs and drives

Behavior

Recovery process

FIGURE 3.3
The recovery processes are optimized by environments that support them. These environments contain physical, psychological, behavioral, and sociocultural elements.

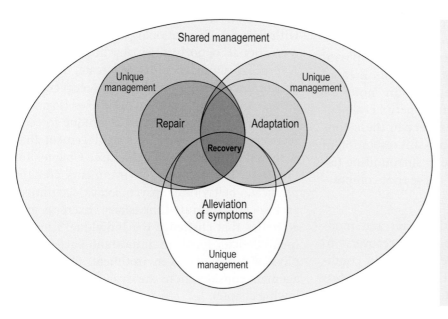

Shared management

Unique management

Unique management

Repair

Adaptation

Recovery

Alleviation of symptoms

Unique management

FIGURE 3.4
Each recovery process has unique management (see Parts 2–4), as well as management that is shared by all three (see Part 5).

MODELING EXERCISE MANAGEMENT ON RECOVERY BEHAVIOR

In a process approach, the management revolves around identifying and supporting behaviors that are considered beneficial to restoring functionality. It is mostly modeled on what humans "do naturally" within their environment to improve their condition, combined with a generous serving of findings from rehabilitation and pain sciences.

The actions or behavior that the individual adopts in their recovery journey can have important implications for its success. When a person is faced with the experience of injury, pain, or loss of functionality they tend to modify their movement behavior. In injury, the role of this specific behavior is to support the underlying physiological process associated with repair, such as reducing weight-bearing activities (behavior) on a sprained ankle (tissue damage and inflammation). This is referred to here as the *protective phase* of the recovery behavior. At a certain point during the repair process, the person will begin to challenge their movement losses. This form of engagement is referred to as the *restorative phase* of the recovery behavior (Fig. 3.5).

Essentially, the exercise management is modeled on these recovery behaviors. It strives

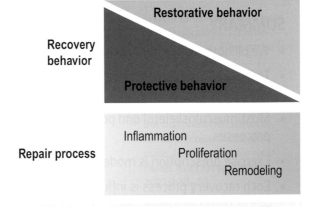

FIGURE 3.5
The recovery behavior consists of a protective phase associated with early stages of repair. In the latter phases, there is a transition to the restorative stage of the recovery behavior, where the individual challenges their movement losses.

to engage the individual in these behaviors, amplifying or attenuating them according to the underlying recovery processes. For example, attenuated movement challenges are used to support the early phases of repair (protective behavior). These challenges can be amplified to support the latter, remodeling, phase of repair (restorative behavior).

36. Järvinen M Healing of a crush injury in rat striated muscle. 4. Effect of early mobilization and immobilization on the tensile properties of gastrocnemius muscle. Acta Chir Scand. 1976;142:47–56.

37. Järvinen M. The effects of early mobilisation and immobilisation on the healing process following muscle injuries. Sports Med. 1993;15:78–89.

38. Goldspink G. Malleability of the motor system: a comparative approach. J Exp Biol. 1985;115:375–91.

39. Montgomery RD. Healing of muscle, ligaments, and tendons. Semin Vet Med Surg (Small Anim). 1989;4:304–11.

40. Kiviranta I, Tammi M, Jurvelin J, Arokoski J, Säämänen AM, Helminen HJ. Articular cartilage thickness and glycosaminoglycan distribution in the young canine knee joint after remobilization of the immobilized limb. J Orthop Res. 1994;12:161–7.

41. Buckwalter JA, Grodzinsky AJ. Loading of healing bone, fibrous tissue, and muscle: implications for orthopaedic practice. J Am Acad Orthop Surg. 1999;7:291–9.

42. Vanwanseele B, Eckstein F, Knecht H, Stussi E, Spaepen A. Knee cartilage of spinal cord-injured patients displays progressive thinning in the absence of normal joint loading and movement. Arthritis Rheum. 2002;46:2073–8.

43. McNulty AL, Guilak F. Mechanobiology of the meniscus. J Biomech. 2015;48: 1469–78.

In this part of the book you will explore how to construct an exercise management for these conditions:

All acute conditions and flareups within the expected time frame of repair, e.g.:
- All acute tissue damage
- Acute pain, whether with/without injury
- Joint and muscle sprains
- Acute low back and neck pain, including disk-related conditions
- Immediate period post-surgery
- Blunt trauma
- Painful phase of frozen shoulder
- Acute tendinopathies
- Acute flareups in persistent pain conditions, e.g. low back and arthritis
- Overuse injuries?

Part 2
Supporting repair

Chapter 4

Contents
Supporting recovery by repair

"I (you) got to move it move it" (with sincere apologies to Reel 2 Real)

Imagine you are in clinic, having to construct an exercise prescription for several patients, all presenting with painful, swollen knees. One has had cruciate ligament surgery, another a knee replacement, and a third a swollen knee which was recently sprained during a sporting activity. All of these conditions have occurred within the last week. What would the exercise advice be? Rest and avoid activities that would stress the joint, or move?

Let's look at this scenario from an evolutionary perspective. Imagine for a minute that it is 5000 BCE and you have just sprained your knee in the wilderness. You are alone and the next human settlement is a week's walking distance away. You are faced with the same dilemma – rest or move. Apart from a short period of immobility, you will soon have to move in search of shelter/protection and forage for food and water. Under these circumstances knee repair would have to resolve within a movement scenario, rather than total rest/immobility (although some rest is useful for repair). From this historical drama we may come to the assumption that the physiology of repair is well adapted to resolve within a dynamic environment. Five thousand years later not much has changed – movement is still the most effective management following acute injuries. Regardless of the underlying condition, all the patients described above would benefit from exercise and activities that involve knee movement rather than immobility. But can we anchor this claim to any science?

The story of movement as a therapeutic modality to support repair took a turn in the 1970s and 1980s. Until that era, most musculoskeletal conditions and post-surgery care were managed by immobilization and extensive periods of bed rest. During that period, several groups of researchers questioned this belief and carried out studies where movement was introduced soon after surgery: mostly within a day or two, but sometimes even before the patient woke up from the operation.[1] It was found that patients who received early mobilization had a shorter hospital stay, less leg edema, less pain and reduced post-operative adhesions. In many of the early studies improvements were seen, even with passive joint mobilization.[2] These findings highlight the beneficial relationship between movement and the biological processes associated with repair.

This chapter will explore the repair process, how it progresses and resolves, and how, using exercise, we can construct an optimal recovery environment (Fig. 4.1). It will also present some very useful management shortcuts.

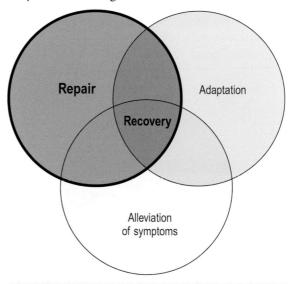

FIGURE 4.1

This part of the book explores functional recovery through supporting repair.

Chapter 4

THE REPAIR PROCESS

A skin laceration, disk prolapse, partial tear of supraspinatus tendon, ankle joint sprain, meniscus damage, bone fracture, and the common cold: seemingly, very different conditions. Yet all share the same physiological restorative mechanisms – the repair process. This innate first aid kit kicks into action immediately when tissue damage is identified anywhere in the body. This remarkable process is responsible for restoring the integrity, structure, and biomechanical and physiological properties of the damaged tissues/organs.

The repair process is the body's healing response to tissue damage in which destroyed tissues are replaced by living tissues.[3] This healing response can be in the form of repair and/ or regeneration. In repair, the original damaged tissue is replaced by a physiologically different scar tissue. This form of tissue healing is seen in skin wounds or ligamentous injuries where the replaced tissue is often biomechanically/physiologically "good enough" but inferior to the original tissues. Regeneration is when the damaged tissue is replaced by the same tissue through proliferation of local tissue or organ-specific cells. This is often seen in muscle injuries where the damaged myocytes can regenerate into fully functioning contractile cells. For the sake of simplicity, these two types of healing events will be broadly referred to as the repair process.

Generally, the repair process follows a similar sequence in all tissues and organs. It is a physiological cascade that is often described as three overlapping stages – *inflammation, proliferation,* and *remodeling* (Fig. 4.2).[4] As will be discussed throughout this and the next chapter, exercise prescription is constructed according to these phases. In order to understand why, how, and when to change the exercise management, we need to take a closer look at the repair process itself.

Phases of repair

The phases of repair are akin to the reconstruction of a collapsed building. The first workers to

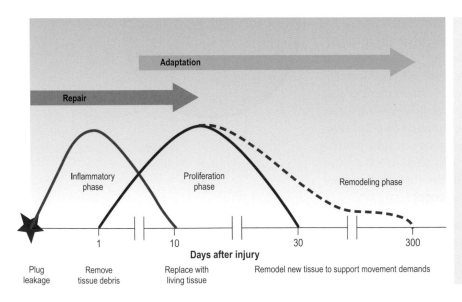

FIGURE 4.2
The three overlapping phases of repair. During inflammation and proliferation, damaged tissue is removed and replaced by living tissue. Note that the latter remodeling phase is an adaptive process.

arrive at the scene seal all the leaks and remove the damage debris. This is largely what happens immediately following injury and during the inflammatory phase. Within moments of tissue damage a blood clot is formed at the site to seal and stop blood leakage. This biological plug is composed of fibrin, platelets, and red blood cells mixed with local cells that actively adhere to each other.[5,6] In the meantime, specialized phagocytic cells (such as neutrophils and macrophages) are activated to seek and clear damaged cells and tissues, remove foreign materials from the wound site, and destroy pathogens in cases of infection.[5,6] The activity of these cells usually peaks in the first 2–3 days after injury.

Subsequently, the initial blood clot transforms into *granulation tissue*, essentially a biological "glue" and "filler" material. It contains the regenerating vascular supply, phagocytic cells, and fibroblasts. The latter are specialized groups of cells which synthesize the collagen fibers which reinforce the granulation tissue. The collagen that is initially deposited forms a weak mesh that has little mechanical strength and can be easily disturbed by vigorous physical activities.

Continuing with the building analogy, during the proliferation phase, a rudimentary scaffolding is erected at the site of damage. At this stage, the granulation tissue is rapidly replaced by connective tissue (scar tissue). This is accompanied by regeneration of the vascular supply, with new buds infiltrating the damaged area. This re-establishes a supply route that provides the nutrients and oxygen that are essential for the synthesis of collagen by the fibroblasts. On the drainage side, new lymphatic islets start to regenerate within the scar to form the initial collecting lymphatics.[7,8] These eventually join to reform the local lymphatic vessels that are needed for removing metabolic and waste products. Generally, the proliferation phase starts within 2–3 days of injury, reaches its peak at about day 14, and continues for about 3–4 weeks.[5,6]

The building site analogy can also be used to illustrate the remodeling phase of repair. When all the emergency work has been carried out (sealing, clearing, gluing, filling, and erecting scaffolding), the initial granulation tissue is progressively replaced by a more permanent and robust connective tissue structure. During this phase there is still a high turnover of collagen, which continues for about 4 months. Thereafter, there is a gradual decrease in the number of fibroblasts and collagen turnover. During remodeling, the tissues are physiologically and morphologically "sculpted" in response to the forces imposed by movement. As will be discussed later, this biological adaptive phenomenon is controlled by a physiological process called *mechanotransduction* (see Chapter 6). In connective tissue the remodeling process may last up to a year or more after injury.[5]

Throughout the proliferation and remodeling phases, there is a progressive increase in the tissue's tensile strength. In animal models, tendon that undergoes surgical repair regains 10% of its original tensile strength within 3 weeks, 20% within 6 weeks, 30% in 9 weeks, and 50% after 12 weeks.[9] So, remodeling in connective tissues is slow. In comparison, muscle damaged by laceration recovers 86% of its tensile strength by 3 weeks and as much as 96% by 2 months.[10] Skin wounds regain around 70% of their tensile strength by 6 weeks (Fig. 4.3). By that point, it is estimated that the person can resume more demanding physical activities.[11] These time scales are highly variable, depending on numerous factors, such as the extent of damage,

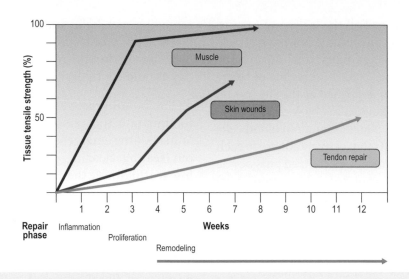

FIGURE 4.3

Tensile strength of muscle, connective tissue, and skin after surgical repair in animals. Clinically, these time scales are highly variable and depend on numerous factors, such as the extent of damage, tissue affected, patient age, and health status. (After Kääriäinen M, Kääriäinen J, Järvinen TL, Sievänen H, Kalimo H, Järvinen M. Correlation between biomechanical and structural changes during the regeneration of skeletal muscle after laceration injury. J Orthop Res. 1998;16:197–206; Gelberman RH, Woo SL-Y, Lothringer K, Akeson WH, Amiel D. Effects of early intermittent passive mobilization on healing canine flexor tendons. J Hand Surg. 1982;7:170–5; and Ireton JE, Unger JG, Rohrich RJ. The role of wound healing and its everyday application in plastic surgery: a practical perspective and systematic review. Plast Reconstr Surg Glob Open. 2013;1:e10–e19.)

surgical procedure, age, health status, and the recovery environment.

REPAIR AND THE INTERSTITIUM

The interstitium caters for the microenvironment supporting the tissue and organ-related cells, such as the myocytes in muscles and fibroblasts in connective tissue. It provides a medium for delivery of nutrients and drainage for metabolic waste products.[12] It is also the place where the drama of inflammation takes place.

The interstitium is arranged as a three-dimensional, sponge-like structure. It consists predominantly of a collagen fiber framework. The spaces within this structure are filled with gel (glycosaminoglycans, GAG) and a variety of cells, such as specialized fibroblasts that service it, and immune cells that patrol and monitor the tissue for invading pathogens or damaged cells.[13] Many components of the interstitial matrix are synthesized by specialized, fibroblast-like, caretaker cells.[14] They synthesize the collagen scaffolding of the matrix itself, the gel (GAG) that fills this space, and the enzymes which remove these components. These caretaker cells are highly responsive to mechanical stimulation and synthesize the matrix's components in response to movement.[15]

Physical activities play an important role in homeostasis and repair of the interstitium. The interstitium contains microchannels that allow the flow of blood filtrate from the capillaries to the initial lymphatics. Similar to a sponge, the interstitium and initial lymphatics are compressible–deformable structures.[14] Flow through this system is influenced by the periodic compression generated in the tissues in which they are embedded; essentially, any event that brings about intermittent tissue deformation (Fig. 4.4). Exercise and movement play an important role in these fluid dynamics.[16] Flow is elevated by the rhythmic contractions of skeletal muscle during exercise (Fig. 4.5), cardiac and arterial pulsations, arteriolar vasomotion, periodic tension in tendons, sliding of fascial planes, skin tension, and so on.[17] Movement facilitates the passage of large protein molecules through the relatively narrow diameter of the interstitial microchannels. During movement, these molecules are "squeezed along" by the intermittent deformation of the tissue, a bit like a peristalsis effect.[12] This flow-enhancing system can be viewed as a *transinterstitial pump.*"

In inflammation, there is an increase in capillary vasodilatation and permeability at the

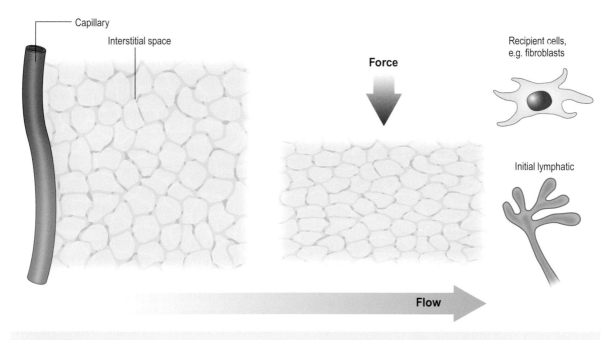

FIGURE 4.4
Flow through the interstitium is enhanced by intermittent forces that deform the tissue. (After Benias PC, Wells RG, Sackey-Aboagye B, Klavan H, Reidy J, Buonocuore D, et al. Structure and distribution of an unrecognized interstitium in human tissues. Sci Rep. 2018;8:4947.)

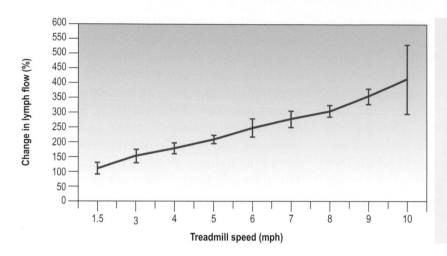

FIGURE 4.5
Lymph flow is elevated by exercise intensity. (After Desai P, Williams AG Jr, Prajapati P, Downey HF. Lymph flow in instrumented dogs varies with exercise intensity. Lymphat Res Biol. 2010;8:143–8.)

site of injury. This causes protein-rich plasma, a blood exudate, to leak into the interstitial space, resulting in raised fluid volume/swelling: edema. Generally, flow through the interstitium is fairly slow but increases ten-fold in inflammation.[12] Edema often has a negative image in physical therapies but it is an essential physiological component of the repair process. It provides a supply and removal "flow highway," enhancing the transport of fluid, nutrients, and macromolecules.[12] It also increases the accessibility of the various repair cells to the site of damage (imagine enlarged, fluid-filled pores in the sponge).

The expanded interstitial fluid space plays an important role in cell communication. Just like on a building site, there is extensive chatter between the different workers directing each other's activities, as well as controlling their movement and location within the building site. Similarly, the interstitial, immune, and parenchymal cells communicate via this expanded fluid medium via the release of a myriad of messenger molecules. These molecules contain biological instructions for all the cellular and vascular processes associated with repair.[13,18]

Through its influences on the transinterstitial pump, movement has several important

roles in supporting the early phases of repair. The elevated flow supports the local increase in metabolic demands by facilitating the supply of nutrients and the removal of inflammatory and metabolic by-products. It also guides the migration and movement of interstitial and immune cells. Movement, through its influence on flow dynamics, helps regulate the swelling in the interstitial space. It limits the accumulation of excessive edema that may otherwise interfere with resolution of inflammation.[19]

Movement also plays a role in guiding the reconstruction of the flow system within the interstitial matrix. Motion stimulates the regeneration, proliferation, and orientation of the capillaries and lymphatic system at the site of repair. With movement, revascularization tends to develop in parallel to the tension forces generated in the tissue (Fig. 4.6A).[20] This vascular organization is well adapted to withstand the physical forces imposed on the tissue.[8] In contrast, following immobilization, vascular regeneration is more disorganized, a formation that tends to fail when movement is reintroduced. The regeneration and reorientation of the lymphatic system within the interstitium are guided by the flow dynamics within this matrix. The precursor lymphatic cells are sensitive to shear

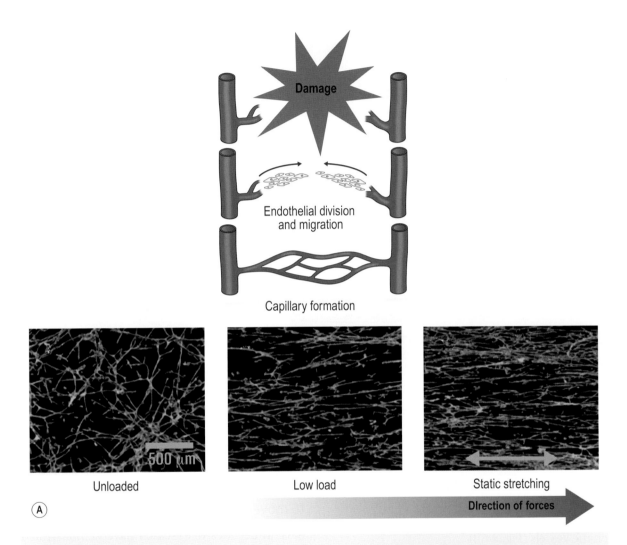

FIGURE 4.6

(A) Reorganisation of the capillary bed after injury is directed by the physical forces imposed on the area by movement, demonstrated in a laboratory sample. In the unloaded model, the capillary bed is disorganized. With low load and static stretching there is progressive microvessel sprouting and organization along the force vectors in the tissue. (After Krishnan L, Underwood CJ, Maas S, Ellis BJ, Kode TC, Hoying JB, et al. Effect of mechanical boundary conditions on orientation of angiogenic microvessels. Cardiovasc Res. 2008;78:324–32.)

Continued

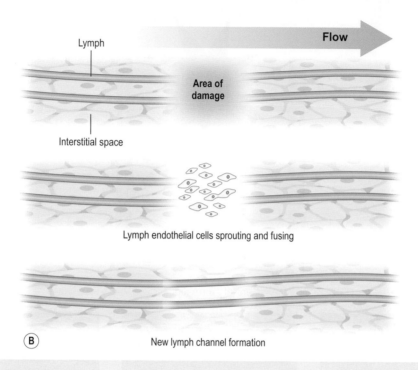

Lymph

Flow

Area of damage

Interstitial space

Lymph endothelial cells sprouting and fusing

(B)　　　　　　New lymph channel formation

FIGURE 4.6 (CONTINUED)

(B) Lymphatic regeneration after injury is guided by fluid flow through the interstitium. (After Boardman KC, Swartz MA. Interstitial flow as a guide for lymphangiogenesis. Circ Res. 2003;92:801–8.)

forces produced by fluid flow across their membranes. In response, they align and proliferate along these fluid vectors to form the new lymphatic vessels (Fig. 4.6B).[7]

MOVEMENT AND REPAIR IN CONNECTIVE TISSUE

Connective tissue, as its name implies, is ubiquitous throughout the body and is damaged in all injuries. Connective tissue injuries can range from minor strains and post-surgical damage to complete tendon and ligament tears or damage to the articular cartilage. Repair in all connective tissues is a fairly similar process that follows the three phases described above.

How connective tissue responds to movement

Several decades of research have demonstrated that moderate loading applied directly to the affected area is essential for connective tissue physiology, morphology, and repair.[21–25] These mechanical stresses can be brought about by functional daily activities and even passive movement, such as in manual therapy.[9,26–32]

Fibroblasts, the builders and caretakers of connective tissues, are highly responsive to movement.[28,33] They continuously "sculpt" the tissues in which they are embedded in response to the forces imposed on them. This sculpting takes place by an ongoing process of adding (synthesis) and removing (degradation) the connective tissue components. On the synthesis side, the fibroblasts produce the precursors for collagen, elastin, and the GAGs, which are then transported into the extracellular space for assembly.[34] The fibroblasts also synthesize the enzymes that degrade and remove unneeded connective tissue components.[35]

Once the collagen has been synthesized and deposited in the extracellular space, it aligns within this matrix along the force vectors generated by movement (Fig. 4.7). This parallel organization endows the tissue with better biomechanical properties, such as tensile strength and extensibility. In the absence of movement, the fibers are randomly deposited within the extracellular space, an organization which results in reduced tensile strength and extensibility (see Chapter 6).[1,36]

Early introduction of movement after injury has been shown to be beneficial for repair in all connective tissues. The tissues display enhanced

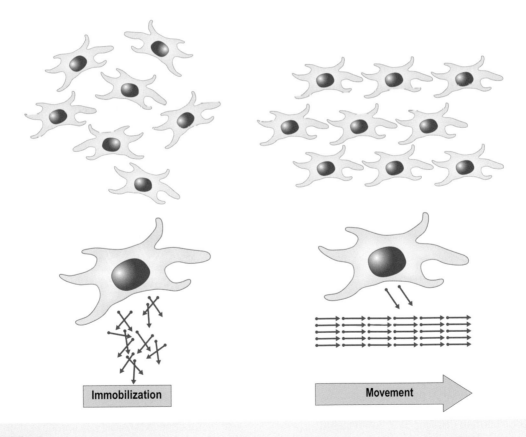

Immobilization

Movement

FIGURE 4.7

Movement directs alignment of the fibroblasts and deposition of collagen along the principal force vectors in the tissue.

45

markers for repair (total DNA and cellularity), higher tensile strength, and normalized stiffness when compared with immobilization (Fig. 4.8), providing that the joint movements are not excessive and scar formation is not disturbed.[37,38] For example, after surgery, tendons that undergo early mobilization tend to fail less often than those immobilized.[39] Early mobilization of the shoulder following arthroscopic rotator cuff repair is safe and results in greater range of movement (ROM) when compared to immobilization protocols.[40] Even in skin, early mobilization of surgical wounds results in scars that closely resemble normal skin.[11,41]

Adhesions and range loss

Lack of movement stimulation has a detrimental influence on ROM. The deposited collagen fibers

are shorter and disorganized, and lack the normal spring-like (crimp) structure that endows connective tissue with an element of extensibility, a bit of "give" when stretched (Fig. 4.9).[1,4]

Further loss of range can come about by collagen fibers sticking to each other through cross-linking (Fig. 4.10).[1,4,42] Collagen is also the body's biological glue, utilized during repair to adhere torn tissues. (In the past, carpenters used collagen to stick furniture together.) Movement improves the balance of GAGs and water content within the tissue, which helps maintain the interfibril distance and lubrication.[1,4] This, in turn, reduces the potential for the collagen fibers to stick to each other and form adhesions (think of spaghetti without the sauce). During immobilization, cross-linking can occur between the fibers themselves or between two gliding surfaces, such as tendons within their sheaths (termed adhesions). The overall effect is a biomechanical loss of movement range. There are other causes

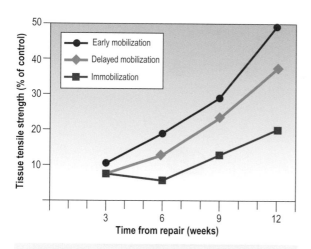

FIGURE 4.8
Tensile strength of repaired tendon after immobilization, delayed mobilization, and early mobilization (using passive motion). (After Gelberman RH, Woo SL-Y, Lothringer K, Akeson WH, Amiel D. Effects of early intermittent passive mobilization on healing canine flexor tendons. J Hand Surg. 1982;7:170–5.)

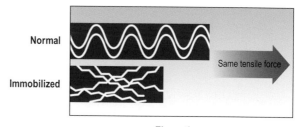

FIGURE 4.9
Movement helps maintain the normal tissue architecture and extensibility. In immobilization, the collagen fibers are disorganized and lose their extensibility, affecting the overall range of movement.

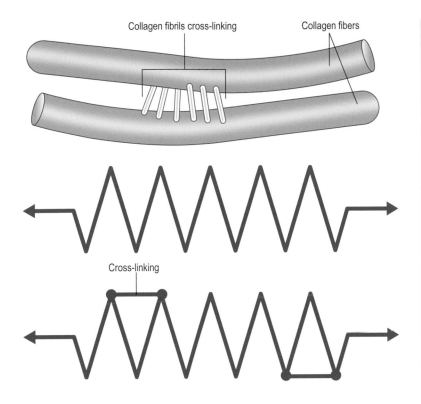

Collagen fibrils cross-linking

Collagen fibers

Cross-linking

FIGURE 4.10
Cross-linking in connective tissue reduces extensibility and contributes to overall loss of range of movement.

of ROM losses related to adaptive and sensitization processes (see Chapters 6 and 10).

Like glue, cross-links tend to "set" (mature) over a period of 1–2 weeks, during which time they increase in their tensile strength and become less malleable to imposed forces.[1,4] Early mobilization during this period can limit this outcome and facilitate ROM recovery.[1,4] Postponing mobilization beyond this window of opportunity can result in a longer rehabilitation period, permanent loss of movement range, and the increased likelihood of a need for manipulation under anesthetic.[1,4] The importance of early mobilization has been demonstrated in post-operative tendon repair. It reduced the excessive proliferation of fibrous tissue and formation of adhesions between the tendon and its sheath.[9,43] Mobilization within 5 days of surgery

resulted in 95% recovery of joint range, 67% if mobilized after 3 weeks, and 19% when mobilized after 12 weeks.[39]

MOVEMENT AND REPAIR IN JOINTS

Essentially, joints are designed to be mobile and operate under repetitive mechanical stresses; therefore, movement plays an important role in their health and during repair. Movement has two principal roles in joint repair. It regulates the homeostatic milieu of the intracapsular space and it has an effect on the repair process in the capsular and intracapsular connective tissue structures.

Synovium and synovial fluid

The physiology of the synovial membrane and fluid and its relationship to the intra-articular structures play an important role in joint repair. The intracapsular space can be imagined as an enlarged "interstitial bubble." Lining this space is the synovium, some 80% of whose surface is cellular and highly vascular. The remaining area, an interstitial space, is a highly permeable matrix that enables the flow of nutrients and drainage between the joint cavity and extracapsular fluid compartments (vascular and lymphatic).[44] The synovial fluid is composed of a blood filtrate/exudate mixed with lubricants produced by specialized synovial cells.[45–47]

One of the main tasks of synovial fluid is to lubricate the joint surfaces and protect them from damage during movement.[48] Synovial fluid also has a role as a physiological medium for the transport of nutrients and for the drainage of the articular cartilage and other intra-articular structures, such as the menisci.[45,46] Chondrocytes, the fibroblast-like cells that service and repair the articular cartilage, have no direct blood supply from the bone below. Their supply of nutrients and drainage of metabolic by-products is dependent solely on transport through the synovial medium.[49] A similar mechanism operates in the avascular portion of the menisci.[48] The supply of nutrients to these areas is carried out partly by diffusion and partly by the pump-like effects of movements on the interstitial space within the cartilage.[22,25,26,50,51]

During physical activities, the synovial fluid is smeared on the articular and intracapsular surfaces, making its contents more accessible to the cartilage cells. The nutrients are then driven through the interstitial space by the intermittent compression of the cartilage/menisci, to reach the target cells.[52] This system is highly sensitive to motion. Even low loading, such as cyclical passive movement, activates this transport mechanism and has been shown to facilitate repair in

articular cartilage. In humans, hyaline cartilage tends to repair by unspecialized, "lower-quality" fibrocartilage. However, more recently it was shown that there may be a limited capacity for hyaline regeneration in the human ankle.[49,53,54]

Interestingly, most tendons have a synovial sheath and synovial fluid. As in joints, this system provides an important nutritional route to the tendon.[55] It has been demonstrated that during active mobilization there is a significant increase in transport of nutrients into the tendon.[56]

The trans-synovial pump

The positive effects of exercise on joint repair are partly attributed to the activation of a physiological mechanism called the *trans-synovial pump*.[45,46] This pump facilitates the formation, flow, and drainage of the synovial fluid contents between the intra-articular compartment and the vascular and lymphatic systems (Fig. 4.11).

The trans-synovial pump has three components that are activated during movement: alternating intra-articular pressures, an increase in synovial membrane blood flow and filtration of exudate into the joint space, and, on the other end, raised drainage into the initial lymphatics (also embedded in the synovial membrane).[45,46] Cyclical repetitive movements, such as walking or cycling, produce varying intra-articular pressures that are related to the joint angle.[57] In the human knee, there is negative (barometric) intra-articular pressure around the neutral angle, associated with flow into the joint space. End-range flexion and extension tend to raise the intra-articular pressure and result in flow out of the joint space.[57,58]

The trans-synovial pump operates in both active and passive movements. Generally, the relationship between the joint angles and flow

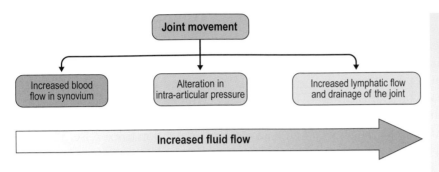

FIGURE 4.11
The trans-synovial pump is activated by movement. During movement, there is an increased flow of nutrients into the joint space and removal of waste products into the initial lymphatics.

patterns are similar in both movement modes; however, pressure and flow rate tend to be elevated during active movement.[59] The intra-articular pressure patterns, and consequently flow rate, vary in different joints and pathologies, such as synovitis, capsulitis, ligament damage, and osteoarthritis.[58–63] Altered biomechanics, such as a damaged anterior cruciate ligament, for example, can also result in altered pressure and flow patterns.[57]

The intracapsular environment in injury

So, what happens to this system in injury? Joint injuries are often associated with damage and inflammation of the synovial lining.[64] The synovial villi swell with an increased flow of exudate (and sometimes blood) into the joint space, in a similar manner to the edema observed in the interstitial space elsewhere. Swelling of the synovium is associated with nociceptive excitation and mechanical encroachment of the villi into the capsular space. This means that, during movement, the sensitive villi could be "pinched" between the articular surfaces, raising the nociceptive barrage and consequently restricting the movement range.[65,66] The joint environment undergoes a physiological change due to an increased metabolic activity of the inflamed synovial lining.[67] This leads to hypoxia and acidosis of the synovial fluid. The combination of these factors can interfere with normal supply and drainage and, consequently, affect the rate and quality of repair of the intra-articular structures.[68]

In articular cartilage, lack of direct mechanical stimulation of the chondrocytes can result in thinning and softening of the articular cartilage, increasing the likelihood of damage.[67,69] This sequence of events can be observed in chronic joint conditions, such as osteoarthritis, where persistent, excessive joint effusion may impair synovial blood flow, alter synovial physiology, and lead ultimately to cartilage damage.[70–74]

Generally, maintaining movement after injury can prevent many of these negative outcomes associated with movement limitations and immobilization. Overall, joint swelling (effusion) and bleeding into the joint space (hemarthrosis) can be controlled through activation of the trans-synovial and interstitial pump by movement.[75,76] Early mobilization of joints using active or passive low loads has been shown to improve the rate and quality of recovery, partly through activation of the trans-synovial pump.[60,77–79] These interventions have often been introduced within 2 days of joint injury or surgery.[76,80] Such loading levels and movement patterns can be emulated by active pendular forms of exercise (see Chapter 14 for demonstration).

Intracapsular adhesions

The synovial membrane seems to be the most sensitive to the effects of disuse/immobilization. Within a few days of immobilization, the synovial villi begin to adhere to each other, resulting in loss of movement range and pain.[81–84] These adhesions are often the earliest cause of range loss after immobilization. The synovial membrane undergoes fibrofatty changes which, in time, proliferate into all the articular soft tissues. In the knee, this proliferation is observed around the cruciate ligament and the undersurface of the quadriceps tendon.[81,82] With the passage of time, the fibrofatty tissue may proliferate to cover the non-articulating area of cartilage.[85] Subsequently, this tissue matures to form adhesions between the two articular surfaces. Such adhesion formation has been shown to occur as early as 15 days after immobilization and to become well established by 30 days.[1,86] Similar changes have been shown to occur in experimental animals and in human facet and knee joints.[87,88] In the knee, similar but less extensive changes have been observed in subjects with damage to the anterior cruciate ligament. Adhesion formation and fibrosis have been found between the patellar fat pad and the synovium adjacent to the damaged ligament.[87]

Importantly for exercise prescription, early mobilization of joints after injury or surgery can help minimize the formation of intra-articular and capsular adhesions.[42] The longer the delay in remobilization, the more likely it is for the adhesion to become less malleable. Generally, adhesions that have already formed during immobilization can be mostly reduced by the return to activity; however, that depends on the extent of the adhesions and tissues involved.

MOVEMENT AND REPAIR IN MUSCLE

Muscle injuries can be differentiated into two groups: sarcomere damage and myofiber tears (Fig. 4.12).[89] Sarcomere damage is observed following unaccustomed or eccentric exercise. These are benign conditions, probably associated with accelerated adaptation to exercise. They are self-limiting and short-lasting (a few days), and do not require any particular care. Often, physical activities can be maintained, even in the presence of pain or discomfort. In muscle tears, the myofibrils rupture and lose their structural continuity. This is often observed at the muscle–tendon junction.

As in other tissues, the repair process in muscle follows a similar pattern comprising inflammation, proliferation, and remodeling phases (Fig. 4.13). Following injury, the loose ends of the ruptured myofibers retract, forming a gap (imagine cutting a stretched rubber band). This gap fills with hematoma and, later, is replaced by granulation tissue (the biological "glue" and "filler"). A seal is formed between the saved ends of the torn myofibers, separating and protecting these stumps from further damage. Within seconds of injury, an inflammatory response is initiated.[90] This process includes immune cell migration and proliferation in the area of damage, reactive vascular changes, and distension of the interstitial space by edema.[91–93] By days 4–6, most of the cellular debris is cleared by the immune cells and the regeneration of muscle fibers can be seen. Subsequently, a scar tissue develops at the site of damage between the loose myofiber ends. Under optimal circumstances, the two ends of the myofiber penetrate the scar tissue to eventually regenerate a continuous myofiber. Introduction of movement within the early phases of repair results in better myofibril regeneration and orientation. Movement also helps the formation of

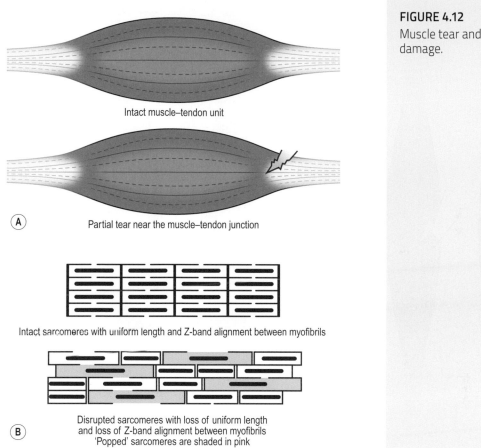

Intact muscle–tendon unit

(A)   Partial tear near the muscle–tendon junction

Intact sarcomeres with uniform length and Z-band alignment between myofibrils

Disrupted sarcomeres with loss of uniform length
and loss of Z-band alignment between myofibrils
(B)   'Popped' sarcomeres are shaded in pink

FIGURE 4.12
Muscle tear and sarcomere damage.

attachments between the myofibers and extracellular collagen matrix.[94–96] This alignment helps optimize the force transmission from the myofiber to its skeletal attachments and expedites the restoration of the muscle's tensile strength.[97]

As regeneration/proliferation progresses, the myotubes mature to become multinucleated muscle cells with their specialized contractile sarcomeres. By this point, the muscle is already entering the remodeling phase. The synthesis and arrangement of the sarcomeres within the recovering myofiber are also influenced by physical activities.[98–100] Depending on the form of activity, sarcomeres can be added serially, lengthways, like links on a chain, or stacked in a parallel arrangement (hypertrophy).[101–102] Generally, movement that contains end-range or speed challenges will drive serial construction of the sarcomeres that culminates in a longer myofiber. Resistance-type activities will result in parallel deposition and increases in force-generating capacity. This activity-specific adaptation will be further discussed in Chapter 7.

The remarkable regenerative capacity of muscle is related to a unique group of specialized stem cells that reside within the muscle, called

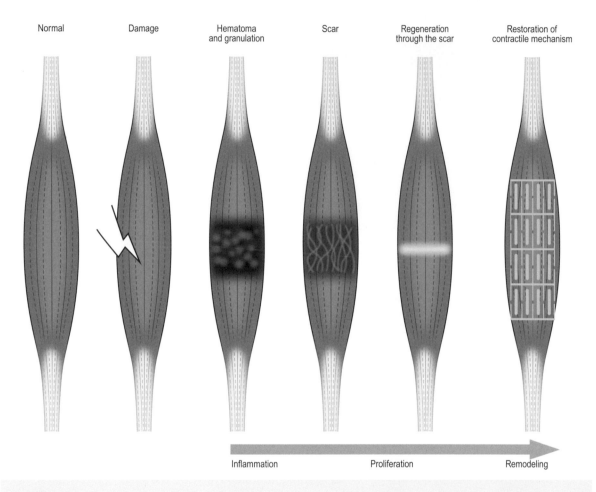

Normal   Damage   Hematoma and granulation   Scar   Regeneration through the scar   Restoration of contractile mechanism

Inflammation   Proliferation   Remodeling

FIGURE 4.13
Repair in muscle.

satellite cells (Fig. 4.14).[103] These stem cells have the capacity to differentiate into fully contractile muscle cells. They are found between the basement membrane and the sarcolemma, and are usually dormant in non-damaged muscle. Within about 2–3 days of injury, these cells are activated and proliferate at the site of damage, to form precursor muscle cells called myoblasts.[91–93] Subsequently, these cells fuse together to form myotubes, each contributing its own nucleus to this precursor of the myofiber. The satellite cells have specialized "feelers" via which they can gauge and respond to physical loading of the muscle. Hence, muscle contraction and movement play an important part in satellite cell differentiation (to myoblasts), formation of myotubes, and their alignment along the force transmission vectors within the muscle.[104–106]

Skeletal muscle has the capacity to regenerate fully without scarring. This outcome is highly dependent on physical activity/movement during all stages of the repair process.[107] This potential for regeneration has been demonstrated in severe fractures where there is extensive damage to the muscle tissue.[108] It is estimated that up to 20% mass loss can be tolerated and recovered by the high regenerative capacity of skeletal muscle. Muscle loss beyond this level can lead to

functional impairment and severe disability.[18] Generally, muscle regeneration completes 3–4 weeks after injury.[109]

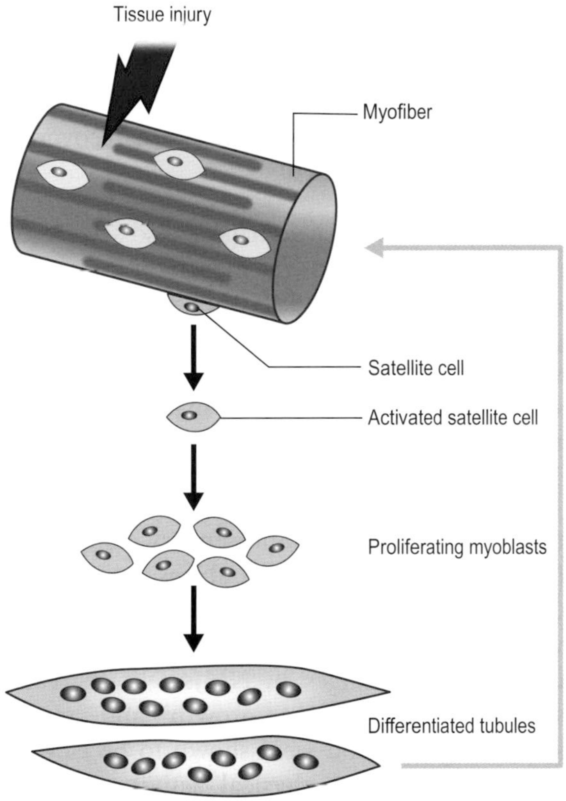

Vascular events during muscle repair

During muscle regeneration, the vascular supply undergoes rapid and profound alterations, with increased capillary numbers, branching, and anastomosis.[110] Within 2 days, there is observable formation of capillaries in the area and a full supply is established by 2–3 weeks.[109] During the early inflammatory phase, this network provides the supply route for the immune cells and delivery of various nutrients required to support the repair process. The rate and intensity of muscle repair are directly correlated with vascular regeneration, especially during the first week post-injury.[97]

Physical activity plays an important role in supporting revascularization. It enhances vascular and lymphatic regeneration and restoration of the interstitial matrix within the muscle.[111,112] In contrast, immobilization brings about significant decreases in capillarization.[97] In animal studies, angiogenesis is initiated within a week of moderate-endurance activity and well-organized capillary networks can be seen after 2 weeks.[113]

In tendons, physical activity promotes a capillary arrangement along the principal force vectors. During repair and remodeling phases, capillaries sprout across from the synovial sheath to the damaged tendon. If mobilization occurs soon after surgery, the vascular supply is restored in a parallel arrangement to the tendon.[114] This organization is adept at withstanding the sliding motion of the tendon within its sheath. However, if the patient is immobilized, the vascular supply tends to sprout at a right angle to the healing tendon; this type of organization tends to fail during remobilization.[114]

FIGURE 4.14
Damaged myofibers are regenerated by the activation of specialized muscle stem cells called satellite cells.

Tissue injury

Myofiber

Satellite cell

Activated satellite cell

Proliferating myoblasts

Differentiated tubules

Lymph flow in instrumented dogs varies with exercise intensity. Lymphat Res Biol. 2010;8:143–8.

17. Schmid-Schönbein GW. Microlymphatics and lymph flow. Physiol Rev. 1990;70:987–1028.

18. Turner MD, Nedjai B, Hurst T, Pennington DJ. Cytokines and chemokines: at the crossroads of cell signalling and inflammatory disease. Biochim Biophys Acta. 2014;1843:2563–82.

19. Villeco JP. Edema: a silent but important factor. J Hand Ther. 2012;25:153–62.

20. Krishnan L, Underwood CJ, Maas S, Ellis BJ, Kode TC, Hoying JB, et al. Effect of mechanical boundary conditions on orientation of angiogenic microvessels. Cardiovasc Res. 2008;78:324–32.

21. Hargens AR, Akeson WH. Stress effects on tissue nutrition and viability. In: Hargens AR, editor. Tissue nutrition and viability. New York: Springer; 1986.

22. Eckstein F, Faber S, Muhlbauer R, Hohe J, Englmeier KH, Reiser M, et al. Functional adaptation of human joints to mechanical stimuli. Osteoarthritis Cartilage 2002;10:44–50.

23. Montgomery RD. Healing of muscle, ligaments, and tendons. Semin Vet Med Surg (Small Anim). 1989;4:304–11.

24. Schild C, Trueb B. Mechanical stress is required for high-level expression of connective tissue growth factor. Exp Cell Res. 2002;274:83–91.

25. Kiviranta I, Jurvelin J, Tammi M, Saamanen AM, Helminen HJ. Weight bearing controls glycosaminoglycan concentration and articular cartilage thickness in the knee joints of young beagle dogs. Arthritis Rheum. 1987;30:801–9.

26. Kiviranta I, Tammi M, Jurvelin J, Arokoski J, Saamanen AM, Helminen HJ. Articular cartilage thickness and glycosaminoglycan distribution in the young canine knee joint after remobilization of the immobilized limb. J Orthop Res. 1994;12:161–7.

27. Buckwalter JA, Grodzinsky AJ. Loading of healing bone, fibrous tissue, and muscle: implications for orthopaedic practice. J Am Acad Orthop Surg. 1999;7:291–9.

28. Zeichen J, van Griensven M, Bosch U. The proliferative response of isolated human tendon fibroblasts to cyclic biaxial mechanical strain. Am J Sports Med 2000;28:888–92.

29. Skutek M, van Griensven M, Zeichen J, Brauer N, Bosch U. Cyclic mechanical stretching enhances secretion of interleukin 6 in human tendon fibroblasts. Knee Surg Sports Traumatol Arthrosc. 2001;9:322–6.

30. Grinnell F, Ho CH. Transforming growth factor beta stimulates fibroblast-collagen matrix contraction by different mechanisms in mechanically loaded and unloaded matrices. Exp Cell Res. 2002;273:248–55.

31. Yamaguchi N, Chiba M, Mitani H. The induction of c-fos mRNA expression by mechanical stress in human periodontal ligament cells. Arch Oral Biol. 200;47:465–71.

32. Bosch U, Zeichen J, Skutek M, Albers I, van Griensven M, Gassler N. Effect of cyclical stretch on matrix synthesis of human patellar tendon cells. Unfallchirurg. 2002;105:437–42.

33. Mudera VC, Pleass R, Eastwood M, Tarnuzzer R, Schultz G, Khaw P, et al. Molecular responses of human dermal fibroblasts to dual cues: contact guidance and mechanical load. Cell Motil Cytoskeleton. 2000;45:1–9.

34. Carlstedt CA, Nordin M. Biomechanics of tendons and ligaments. In: Nordin M, Frankel VH, editors. Basic biomechanics of the musculoskeletal system. London: Lea & Febiger; 1989. Ch. 3, pp. 698–738.

35. Bauer EA, Stricklin GP, Jeffrey JJ, Eisen AZ. Collagenase production by human skin fibroblasts. Biochem Biophys Res Comm. 1975;64:232–40.

36. Gelberman RH, Amifl D, Gonsalves M, Woo S, Akeson WH. The influence of protected passive mobilization on the healing of flexor tendons: a biochemical and microangiographic study. Hand. 1981;13:120–8.

37. Viidik A. Interdependence between structure and function in collagenous tissues. In: Viidik A, Vuust J, editors. Biology of collagen. London: Academic Press; 1980. pp. 257–80.

38. Vailas AC, Tipton CM, Matthes RD, Gart M. Physical activity and its influence on the repair process of medial collateral ligaments. Connect Tissue Res. 1981;9:25–31.

39. Strickland JW, Glogovac V. Digital function following flexor tendon repair in zone 2: a comparison of immobilization

and controlled passive motion techniques. J Hand Surg. 1980;5:537–43.

40. Shen C, Tang ZH, Hu JZ, Zou GY, Xiao RC, Yan DX. Does immobilization after arthroscopic rotator cuff repair increase tendon healing? A systematic review and meta-analysis. Arch Orthop Trauma Surg. 2014;134:1279–85.

41. Lagrana NA, Alexander H, Strauchler I, Mehta A, Ricci J. Effect of mechanical load in wound healing. Ann Plast Surg. 1983;10:200–8.

42. Akeson WH, Amiel D, Mechanic GL, Woo SL-Y, Harwood FL, Hamer ML. Collagen cross-linking alterations in joint contractures: changes in the reducible cross-links in periarticular connective tissue collagen after nine weeks of immobilization. Connect Tissue Res. 1977;5:15–19.

43. Woo SL, Gelberman RH, Cobb NG, Amiel D, Lotheringer K, Akeson WH. The importance of controlled passive mobilization on flexor tendon healing. Acta Orthop Scand. 1981;52:615–22.

44. Knight AD, Levick JR. The density and distribution of capillaries around a synovial cavity. Q J Exp Physiol. 1983;68:629–44.

45. Levick JR. Synovial fluid and trans–synovial flow in stationary and moving normal joints. In: Helminen HJ, Kivaranki I, Tammi M, editors. Joint loading: biology and health of articular structures. Bristol: John Wright; 1987. pp. 149–86.

46. Levick JR. Microvascular architecture and exchange in synovial joints. Microcirculation 1995;2:217–33.

47. Scott D, Coleman PJ, Mason RM, Levick JR. Direct evidence for the partial reflection of hyaluronan molecules by the lining of rabbit knee joints during trans-synovial flow. J Physiol. 1998;508:619–23.

48. Fox AJS, Bedi A, Rodeo SA. The basic science of human knee menisci structure, composition, and function. Sports Health. 2012;4:340–51.

49. Gershuni DH, Hargens AR, Danzig LA. Regional nutrition and cellularity of the meniscus. Implications for tear and repair. Sports Med. 1988;5:322–7.

50. Vanwanseele B, Eckstein F, Knecht H, Stussi E, Spaepen A. Knee cartilage of spinal cord-injured patients displays progressive thinning in the absence of normal joint loading and movement. Arthritis Rheum. 2002;46:2073–8.

51. Chang JK, Ho ML, Lin SY. Effects of compressive loading on articular cartilage repair of knee joint in rats. Kaohsiung J Med Sci. 1996;12:453–60.

52. Maroudas A. Distribution and diffusion of solutes in articular cartilage. Biophys J. 1970:10.

53. Hsueh M-F, Önnerfjord P, Bolognesi MP, Easley ME, Kraus VB. Analysis of "old" proteins unmasks dynamic gradient of cartilage turnover in human limbs. Science Advances. 2019;5:eaax3203.

54. Knapik DM, Harris JD, Pangrazzi G, Griesser MJ, Siston RA, Agarwal S, et al. The basic science of continuous passive motion in promoting knee health: a systematic review of studies in a rabbit model. Arthroscopy. 2013;29:1722–31.

55. Fenwick SA, Hazleman BL, Riley GP. The vasculature and its role in the damaged and healing tendon. Arthritis Res Ther. 2002;4:252.

56. Lundborg G, Holm S, Myrhage R. The role of the synovial fluid and tendon sheath for flexor tendon nutrition. Scand J Plast Reconstr Surg. 1980;14:99–107.

57. Pedowitz RA, Gershuni DH, Crenshaw AG, Petras SL, Danzig LA, Hargens AR. Intraarticular pressure during continuous passive motion of the human knee. J Orthop Res. 1989;7:530–7.

58. Alexander C, Caughey D, Withy S, Van Puymbroeck E, Munoz D. Relation between flexion angle and intraarticular pressure during active and passive movement of the normal knee. J Rheumatol. 1996;23:889–95.

59. Wood L, Ferrell WR, Baxendale RH. Pressures in normal and acutely distended human knee joints and effects on quadriceps maximal voluntary contractions. Q J Exp Physiol. 1988;73:305–14.

60. Strand E, Martin GS, Crawford MP, Kamerling SG, Burba DJ. Intra-articular pressure, elastance and range of motion in healthy and injured racehorse metacarpophalangeal joints. Equine Vet J. 1998;30:520–7.

61. Goddard NJ, Gosling PT. Intra-articular fluid pressure and pain in osteoarthritis of the hip. J Bone Joint Surg Br. 1988;70:52–5.

62. Hashimoto T, Suzuki K, Nobuhara K. Dynamic analysis of intraarticular pressure in the glenohumeral joint. J Shoulder Elbow Surg. 1995;4:209–18.

63. Jensen K, Graf BK. The effects of knee effusion on quadriceps strength and knee intra-articular pressure. Arthroscopy. 1993;9:52–6.

64. Swärd P, Frobell R, Englund M, Roos H, Struglics A. Cartilage and bone markers and inflammatory cytokines are increased in synovial fluid in the acute phase of knee injury (hemarthrosis): a cross-sectional analysis. Osteoarthritis Cartilage. 2012;20:1302–8.

65. Ahlqvist J. Swelling of synovial joints – an anatomical, physiological and energy metabolical approach. Pathophysiol. 2000;7:1–19.

66. Shay AK, Bliven ML, Scampoli DN, Otterness IG, Milici AJ. Effects of exercise on synovium and cartilage from normal and inflamed knees. Rheumatol Int. 1995;14:183–9.

67. Haapala J, Arokoski JP, Ronkko S, Agren U, Kosma VM, Lohmander LS, et al. Decline after immobilisation and recovery after remobilisation of synovial fluid IL1, TIMP, and chondroitin sulphate levels in young beagle dogs. Ann Rheum Dis. 2001;60:55–60.

68. Fassbender HG. Significance of endogenous and exogenous mechanisms in the development of osteoarthritis. In: Helminen HJ, editor. Joint loading: biology and health of articular structures. Bristol: John Wright; 1987.

69. Vincent TL, Wann AK. Mechanoadaptation: articular cartilage through thick and thin. J Physiol. 2019;597:1271–81.

70. Levick JR. Hypoxia and acidosis in chronic inflammatory arthritis; relation to vascular supply and dynamic effusion pressure. J Rheumatol. 1990;17:579–82.

71. James MJ, Cleland LG, Rofe AM, Leslie AL. Intraarticular pressure and the relationship between synovial perfusion and metabolic demand. J Rheumatol. 1990;17:521–7.

72. Hardy J, Bertone AL, Muir WW. Joint pressure influences synovial tissue blood flow as determined by colored microspheres. J Appl Physiol. 1996;80:1225–32.

73. Geborek P, Moritz U, Wollheim FA. Joint capsular stiffness in knee arthritis. Relationship to intraarticular volume, hydrostatic pressures, and extensor muscle function. J Rheumatol. 1989;16:1351–8.

74. Vegter J, Klopper PJ. Effects of intracapsular hyperpressure on femoral head blood flow. Laser Doppler flowmetry in dogs. Acta Orthop Scand. 1991;64:337–41.

75. O'Driscoll SW, Kumar A, Salter RB. The effect of continuous passive motion on the clearance of a hemarthrosis from a synovial joint. An experimental investigation in the rabbit. Clin Orthop Relat Res. 1983;(176):305–11.

76. James MJ, Cleland LG, Gaffney RD, Proudman SM, Chatterton BE. Effect of exercise on 99mTc-DTPA clearance from knees with effusions. J Rheumatol. 1994;21:501–4.

77. Greene WB. Use of continuous passive slow motion in the postoperative rehabilitation of difficult pediatric knee and elbow problems. J Pediatr Orthop. 1983;3:419–23.

78. Simkin PA, de Lateur BJ, Alquist AD, Questad KA, Beardsley RM, Esselman PC. Continuous passive motion for osteoarthritis of the hip: a pilot study. Rheumatol. 1999;26:1987–91.

79. Raab MG, Rzeszutko D, O'Connor W, Greatting MD. Early results of continuous passive motion after rotator cuff repair: a prospective, randomized, blinded, controlled study. Am J Orthop. 1996;25:214–20.

80. Noyes FR, Mangine RE, Barber S. Early knee motion after open and arthroscopic anterior cruciate ligament reconstruction. Am J Sports Med. 1987;15:149–60.

81. Trudel G, Seki M, Uhthoff HK. Synovial adhesions are more important than pannus proliferation in the pathogenesis of knee joint contracture after immobilization: an experimental investigation in the rat. J Rheumatol. 2000;27:351–7.

82. Trudel G, Jabi M, Uhthoff HK. Localized and adaptive synoviocyte proliferation characteristics in rat knee joint contractures secondary to immobility. Arch Phys Med Rehabil. 2003;84:1350–6.

83. Ando A, Hagiwara Y, Onoda Y, Hatori K, Suda H, Chimoto E, et al. Distribution of type A and B synoviocytes in the adhesive and shortened synovial membrane during immobilization of

the knee joint in rats. Tohoku J Exp Med. 2010;221:161–8.

84. Matsumoto F, Trudel G, Uhthoff HK. High collagen type I and low collagen type III levels in knee joint contracture: an immunohistochemical study with histological correlate. Acta Orthop Scand. 2002;73:335–43.

85. Akeson WH, Amiel D, Abel MF, Garfin SR, Woo SL. Effects of immobilization on joints. Clin Orthop Relat Res. 1987;(219):28–37.

86. Evans EB, Eggers GWN, Butler JK, Blumel J. Experimental immobilisation and remobilisation of rat knee joints. J Bone Joint Surg. 1960;42:737–58.

87. Finsterbush A, Frankl U, Mann G. Fat pad adhesion to partially torn anterior cruciate ligament: a cause of knee locking. Am J Sports Med. 1989;17:92–5.

88. Enneking WF, Horowitz M. The intra-articular effect of immobilization on the human knee. J Bone Joint Surg. 1972;54:973–85.

89. McHugh MP, Tyler TF. Muscle strain injury vs muscle damage: two mutually exclusive clinical entities. Transl Sports Med. 2019;2:102–8.

90. Yang W, Hu P. Skeletal muscle regeneration is modulated by inflammation. J Orthop Transl. 2018;13:25–32.

91. Kharraz Y, Guerra J, Mann CJ, Serrano AL, Muñoz-Cánoves P. Macrophage plasticity and the role of inflammation in skeletal muscle repair. Mediators Inflamm. 2013;2013:491497.

92. Rigamonti E, Zordan P, Sciorati C, Rovere-Querini P, Brunelli S. Macrophage plasticity in skeletal muscle repair. Biomed Res Int. 2014;2014:560629.

93. Tidball JG, Villalta SA. Regulatory interactions between muscle and the immune system during muscle regeneration. Am J Physiol Regul Integr Comp Physiol. 2010;298: R1173–87.

94. Järvinen MJ, Lehto MU. Healing of a crush injury in rat striated muscle. 2. A histological study of the effect of early mobilization and immobilization on the repair processes. Acta Pathol Microbiol Scand. 1975;83:269–82.

95. Järvinen M. Healing of a crush injury in rat striated muscle. 4. Effect of early mobilization and immobilization on the tensile properties of gastrocnemius muscle. Acta Chir Scand. 1976;142:47–56.

96. Järvinen M. 1993 The effects of early mobilisation and immobilisation on the healing process following muscle injuries. Sports Med. 1993;15:78-89.

97. Järvinen M. Healing of a crush injury in rat striated muscle. 3. A micro-angiographical study of the effect of early mobilization and immobilization on capillary ingrowth. Acta Pathol Microbiol Scand. 1976;84:85–94.

98. Baldwin KM, Haddad F. Skeletal muscle plasticity: cellular and molecular responses to altered physical activity paradigms. Am J Phys Med Rehabil. 2002;81:S40–51.

99. Baker JH, Matsumoto DE. Adaptation of skeletal muscle to immobilization in a shortened position. Muscle Nerve. 1988;11:231–44.

100. Goldspink G. Changes in muscle mass and phenotype and the expression of autocrine and systemic growth factors by muscle in response to stretch and overload. J Anat. 1999;194:323–34.

101. Williams PE, Goldspink G. Changes in sarcomere length and physiological properties in immobilized muscle. J Anat. 1978;127(Pt 3):459–68.

102. Tabary JC, Tabary C, Tardieu C, Tardieu G, Goldspink G. Physiological and structural changes in the cat's soleus muscle due to immobilization at different lengths by plaster casts. J Physiol. 1972;224:231–44.

103. Mukund K, Subramaniam S. Skeletal muscle: a review of molecular structure and function, in health and disease. Wiley Interdiscip Rev Syst Biol Med. 2020;12:e1462.

104. Roth SM, Martel GF, Ivey FM, Lemmer JT, Tracy BL, Metter EJ, et al. Skeletal muscle satellite cell characteristics in young and older men and women after heavy resistance strength training. J Gerontol A Biol Sci Med Sci. 2001;56:B240–7.

105. Trappmann B, Gautrot JE, Connelly JT, Strange DG, Li Y, Oyen ML, et al. Extracellular-matrix tethering regulates stem-cell fate. Nat Mater. 2012;11:642–9.

106. Allbrook DB, Baker W deC, Kirkaldy-Willis WH. Muscle regeneration in experimental animals and in man. J Bone Joint Surg. 1966;48B:153–69.

107. Greising SM, Warren GL, Southern WM, Nichenko AS, Qualls AE, Corona BT. Early rehabilitation for volumetric muscle loss injury augments endogenous regenerative

Chapter 5

Contents
Exercise prescription supporting repair

This chapter will explore how to construct an exercise management during the first weeks of the repair process, i.e., how we can support and enrich the repair environment.

From the vast research conducted over several decades, it has become clear that movement has an essential role in optimizing tissue repair. There is nothing in medical science that matches the extensive beneficial effects that movement has on supporting repair and return to functionality. Movement encourages the activation of the transinterstitial and trans-synovial pump systems and supports tissue nutrition and drainage during a period of heightened regenerative and metabolic activity. Movement plays an important role in guiding the regeneration of capillaries and restoration of the lymphatic system at the site of damage. It directs the synthesis of connective tissue components by fibroblasts and their deposition within the connective and interstitial tissues. In muscle, movement helps in the differentiation of satellite cells into myotubes and the subsequent restoration of the myofibers: their orientation within the whole muscle, attachments to the extracellular matrix, and anchorage to the muscle's fascia and tendons. There is also evidence that peripheral nerve regeneration is enhanced by physical activities. To this long list of benefits, we need to add the reduced potential for adhesion formation in tissues that have healed under mobilization, the maintenance of undamaged tissue, and the general health and well-being of the individual. With movement, the overall outcome is tissues which have closer morphological, biomechanical, and physiological properties to the original tissue: properties that are well adapted to support the demands of functional activities.

In contrast, immobilization and withdrawal from physical activity can result in negative outcomes for the repair process. These include prolonged duration and lower quality of repair, and atrophy of damaged and saved tissues. It also impacts the tissues' biomechanical properties, resulting in decreased tensile strength and loss of extensibility and range of movement (ROM). Immobility may prolong and increase levels of pain, and ultimately, delay return to, and reduce, the individual's functional capacity.

Often, the main reason for excessive rest and immobility after injury may relate to patients' and therapists' fears of tissue re-damage and exacerbation of pain. On the majority of occasions, these fears do not correlate with research findings demonstrating that movement is more likely to support, enhance, and expedite the repair process. Mostly, research demonstrates that tissue repair within a dynamic environment results in greater strength gains than under immobilization. Hence, the possibility that early mobilization will curtail repair is very low; however, re-damage and pain are always potential outcomes. These issues can be resolved by activity grading strategies, as discussed in Chapter 9.

FEATURES OF EXERCISE DURING REPAIR

So far, it has been established that the repair process can be supported by physical activities. This raises the question of which form of exercise would be beneficial during the different stages of repair. Should we prescribe functional or extra-functional exercise, or both? This decision is guided by the prevailing physiological processes during the three phases of repair.

Management in the inflammatory and proliferation phases is largely similar (loosely termed the early phase of repair). It aims to create an optimal milieu for tissue healing and proliferation, and to regulate edema and joint effusion. This effect can be achieved by exercise that generates intermittent compression of the affected tissue and cyclical movement of joints; in essence, the focus is to engage the transinterstitial and trans-synovial pump systems. Both functional and extra-functional exercise approaches can be used to produce these effects, as long as they are:

- applied locally to the affected tissues/joints
- cyclical in nature
- performed in ranges and at loading levels that support tissue repair processes.

These principles can be demonstrated in an acute knee sprain. Extra-functional challenges could include gentle, low-loading, cyclical movement in standing, sitting, or lying down. These can be in the form of pendular movements applied directly to the affected area; see Chapter 14 for an exercise demonstration applied to major areas/joints of the body. Using a functional exercise approach may be more achievable for the patient, as many of these physiological movement patterns can be readily induced by and integrated into daily activities (such as walking). Probably a mixture of the two approaches may be useful in the early phases – in particular, if the individual is unable to execute full functional activities, such as walking. In this case, the limited walking can be supported with extra-functional pendular knee movements in sitting; see Chapter 14 for knee and hip (Figs 14.12A–B, 14.13A–E, and 14.24A–D, and for shoulder (Figs 14.4A–G).

The management aims and exercise approach change as the repair process enters the remodeling phase (loosely termed the latter phase of repair). During this stage, the tissues are adapting specifically to the imposed physical environment (related to the movement behavior of the individual). Here, management aims to guide tissue remodeling/adaptation that is biomechanically

and physiologically attuned to support functional activities. At this point, there is a shift in management towards functional movement challenges by gradually amplifying daily activities (see Chapter 9). Generally, an extra-functional exercise approach is unlikely to provide meaningful benefits during the remodeling phase. Extra-functional activities are often "sub-physiological," providing loading forces and exposure durations that are below those generated by daily activities (see Chapter 2). Hence, they should be rapidly superseded by functional challenges.

WAIT WITH THE STRETCHING! BUT MOVE IT

During the early phase of repair, the experience of stiffness and ROM loss is associated with tissue swelling and stretch sensitivity, which is a central nervous system process (see Chapter 12). Often, the individual will try to alleviate these symptoms by stretching. However, stretching is unnecessary and may even be detrimental for recovery at the onset of the repair process. During this phase, the newly formed fibers have a low tensile strength and could be re-damaged by the forces of stretching. Additionally, stretching is largely ineffective at activating the transinterstitial and trans-synovial pumps, which are needed in order to reduce tissue swelling. Instead of stretching, active movement within tolerable ranges can be used to stimulate the tissue pumps (transinterstitial and trans-synovial). This can help manage the swelling and consequently alleviate the symptoms of stiffness (see Chapter 12).

SUMMARY OF PART 2: SUPPORTING REPAIR

The conditions associated with recovery by repair and principles for their management by exercise/physical activities are listed in the summary table below (see examples in Chapter 14).

Condition	All acute conditions and flareups within the expected time frame of repair, e.g.:
	All acute tissue damage
	Acute pain, whether with/without injury
	Joint and muscle sprains
	Acute low back and neck pain, including disk-related conditions
	Immediate period post-surgery
	Blunt trauma
	Painful phase of frozen shoulder
	Acute tendinopathies
	Acute flareups in persistent pain conditions, e.g. low back and arthritis
	Overuse injuries?
Recovery process	**Repair**
Specific management	Cyclical and repetitive loading
	Applied locally to affected area
	Initially, movement can be fragmented to specific joints
	Active or passive movement
	Any movement pattern but preferably functional; extra-functional is OK but should be rapidly replaced by functional activities
	Tolerable discomfort/pain-free movement
	Activity grading: initially, may need attenuation to sub-functional intensities and then amplification to low or moderate functional loading

In this part of the book, you will explore how to construct an exercise management plan for these conditions:

All conditions affecting functional capacity and control of performance (not necessarily associated with repair or pain):
- Conditions affecting the skillful performance of activities
- Conditions affecting task components (force, endurance, speed and range of movement, balance, and coordination)
- Remodeling phase of repair
- Restorative phase post-surgery
- Conditions in which inducing structural/biomechanical change is recommended for recovery
- Post-immobilization movement deficits such as range of movement loss
- Stiff phase of frozen shoulder
- Musculoskeletal effects of detraining
- Motor control deficits due to central nervous system damage
- Postural and movement re-education/rehabilitation

Part 3
Supporting adaptation

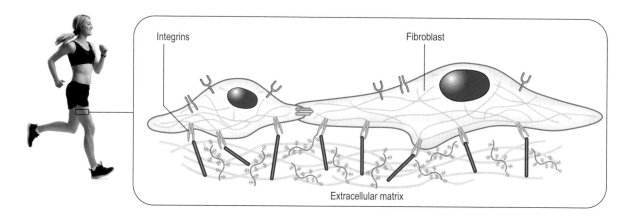

FIGURE 6.3

Fibroblasts (and myocytes) can detect tension across their membranes via specialized molecules on their surface. One such "feeler" is integrin, which projects from the membrane and attaches to the extracellular matrix. Integrins transmit information about movement to the cell's nucleus, which in turn synthesizes a range of connective tissue components (such as collagen). These "materials" are transported to be assembled in the extracellular matrix.

This, in turn, initiates a cascade of molecular events that culminate in synthesis of the various tissue-specific components, as well as the enzymes that remove them.

Fibrobast "relatives": Fibroblasts have several "relatives" in other connective tissues that share the capacity for mechanotransduction: tenocytes in tendon, chondrocytes in articular cartilage, and osteoblasts in bone. They all play a role in maintaining structure, function, and repair within their respective tissues.[12]

Mechanotransduction is the physiological mechanism behind adaptive tissue recovery that is seen in remedial activities, as well as negative dysfunctional changes, such as those observed post-immobilization or in detraining. Underloading the tissues (physical event) modifies the mechanical microenvironment of the mechanocytes and, through mechanotransduction, results in tissue atrophy (biological event).

Many of these negative changes can be prevented and reversed, to varying degrees, by maintaining or elevating the level of activity. These movement challenges will stimulate mechanotransduction and drive the adaptive reorganization needed to support functional demands (Fig. 6.4).

Adaptation in connective tissue and articular structures

In connective tissue, loading stimulates the fibroblasts to synthesize the materials that constitute the tissue's structure and function, including the collagen fibers, the gel between the fibers, and even the enzymes that remove collagen. Additionally, mechanotransduction has an important role in the deposition and arrangement of the collagen in the extracellular matrix. Mechanical stimulation directs the alignment of the fibroblasts and the arrangement of collagen fibers in the matrix along the direction of the principal strains.[10,11] This arrangement contributes in part to the tissue's tensile strength and extensibility.

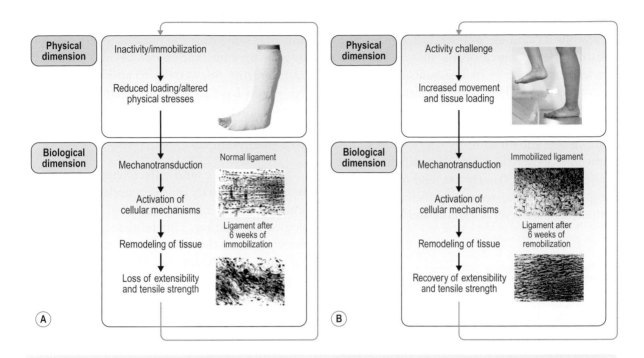

FIGURE 6.4

(A) Mechanotransduction in adaptation to injury, immobility, and inactivity. (B) Mechanotransduction and functional recovery.

Environmental conditions in which physical challenges are reduced below functional levels (sub-functional/underloading) have detrimental effects on the structure, physiology, and biomechanics of connective tissues. These include abnormal cross-linking and adhesion, as well as changes in the size and orientation of the collagen fibers. The outcome is decreased tissue extensibility, increased stiffness, loss of tensile strength, and range limitation that ultimately impact functional capacity (see Chapter 4 for further discussion).[3,13–25]

Adaptive recovery in connective tissues

Mechanotransduction plays an important role during remobilization or training. Physical challenges can help reverse many of the dysfunctional changes with varying degrees of success, depending on factors such as the duration of immobilization, extent of adhesions, age, length of time between immobilization and remobilization, and quality of environmental challenges, to name but a few.

Reintroducing movement challenges supports the recovery of the tissues' biomechanical and physiological properties. This takes place through normalization of the gel content, reduction of abnormal collagen cross-links, remodeling of the crimp structure, normalization of fiber reorientation, and reduction of adhesions.[3,26] Remobilization has been shown to improve the tissue's tensile strength by helping to restore its unique architecture and by compacting the collagen fibrils into thicker and denser bundles.[3,26–30] In ligaments, reorganization of collagen fibers can take place in as little as 6 weeks of remobilization. In laboratory studies, collagen that underwent recurrent tension loading was shown to be 10 times stronger and eight-fold denser than non-stimulated bundles.[5] Generally, connective tissues tend to adapt over long time periods, regaining their mechanical properties over several months and longer.[3,23]

> **Management implications:** After injury or surgery there is a 1–2-week window of opportunity to reduce the potential for adhesion formation. Adhesions have low tensile strength in the first 2 weeks of their formation before the cross-links fully mature and set. During this period, their development can be minimized by normal movement or activity. However, once they mature, they can sometimes have the consistency of a tough leather belt! At this point it will require greater effort and lengthy management to recover the tissues' extensibility/ROM, so keep them moving early on after surgery or injury.

Muscle adaptation

Imagine an unusual situation where you changed an exercise routine over several months, starting, say, with yoga, then 6 months later switching to weight training, then to sprint running and sometime later to long-distance running. Your muscles would have to undergo dramatic transformation in order to support you optimally in these varied activities. Broadly speaking, yoga may require some muscle groups to undergo length change; weightlifting results in force generation change; sprint running requires force

production at high velocities; and long-distance running transforms the muscles' energy supply, favoring an endurance mode. As you switch the training from one activity to another, the muscles would have to adapt to operate at varying forces, velocities, movement ranges, and durations, while keeping in check the efficiency of their energy supply.

The efficiency and effectiveness of movement depend partly on the muscles' capacity to undergo the extensive morphological and physiological adaptation. This reorganization can be observed from the molecular level to gross visual changes in the muscle's size and shape; from transcription events within cells' nuclei (coding for vital functions of the myocytes), synthesis of actin and myosin contractile protein and arrangement of the sarcomere (contractile apparatus), and alteration in mitochondrial activity (energy supply system), along with changes in the extracellular matrix (providing structural and biochemical support), and reorganization of blood supply (oxygen and nutrients) and lymphatic drainage (for metabolic byproducts).[31] How, then, does the muscle adapt specifically to generate more force or operate at different lengths, velocities, and energy requirements?

Force adaptation

Long-term changes in force generation are related to the number of parallel sarcomeres within the muscle fiber.[32] Depending on the nature of the movement demand, sarcomeres can be added or removed, either in parallel or serially (i.e., "bulky" or "lean and long" muscle, Fig. 6.5). Recurrent activities that require increases in force generation result in the synthesis of actin and myosin contractile proteins. These, in turn, are assembled into sarcomeres, which are subsequently arranged in parallel within the muscle

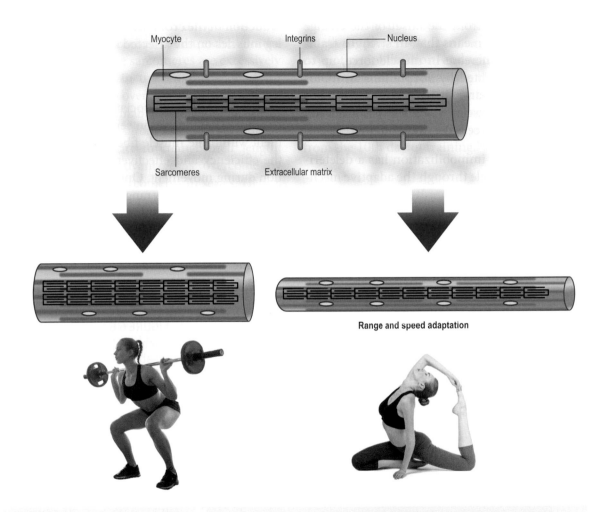

FIGURE 6.5
Mechanotransduction plays an important role in directing the arrangement of sarcomeres in muscle in response to physical activities. For force, sarcomeres are added in parallel; for speed and range, they are added serially. These adaptations can be combined, depending on the type of activities in which the individual participates, and are specific to that person's principal activity/training.

fiber (hypertrophy).[32] This process starts soon after demanding physical activity. The precursory processes that lead to the production of the contractile proteins are already evident in the muscle's nuclei within 1 hour of exercising, and still observable 48 hours later.[33] The formation of new sarcomeres can be observed 4 days after exercising the muscle[34] (which means that we bulk up after and not during exercise). Generally, muscle hypertrophy or atrophy occurs at

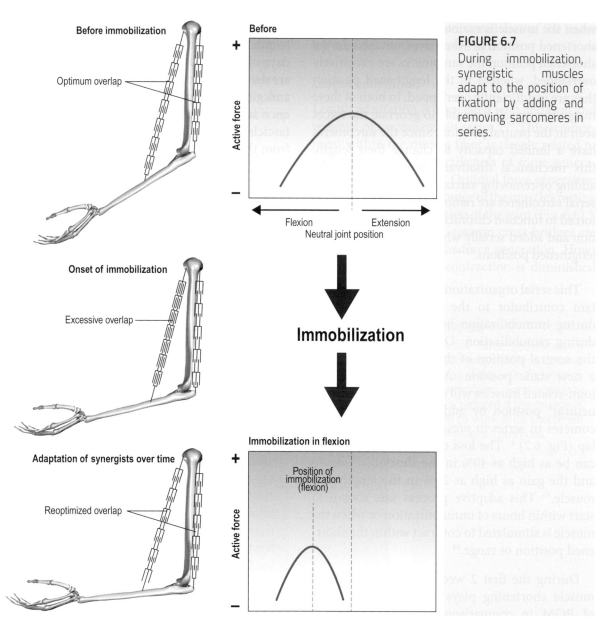

FIGURE 6.7
During immobilization, synergistic muscles adapt to the position of fixation by adding and removing sarcomeres in series.

tend to have a greater fascicle length of the leg muscles when compared with distance runners.[39]

Endurance, energy, and vascular supply

Different physical activities require specific energy provision for optimal muscle perfor-

mance. Mitochondria are the powerhouses of cells, generating most of the energy needed to power the cell's biochemical reactions. These cell organelles are highly adaptive and can alter their volume, structure, and function in response to exercise, disuse, aging, and disease.[51,52] During exercise, there is a rise in molecular stress signals that direct mitochondrial biogenesis and degradation, as well as removal of damaged mitochondria. Endurance activities tend to increase or maintain a high level of mitochondrial content within skeletal muscle, whereas disuse and aging are associated with dysregulation of the mitochondrial networks and impaired function.[51] These mitochondrial changes could partly explain the experience of localized muscle fatigue often seen after injury and immobilization (although there is a large CNS component in the experience of fatigue).

Whether a person is untrained, takes up a new sporting activity, or is a sprinter or a marathon runner will have a profound influence on the blood supply to their muscles. To support the unique nutritional and metabolic demands, muscle blood flow capacity is adapted through a mixture of angiogenesis and altered control of vascular resistance.[53] This adaptation is specific to the principal activity of the individual. For example, distance runners have greater capillary density in their leg muscles in comparison to sprint runners.[54]

Muscle connective tissue and tendon adaptation

Normal mechanical links between the muscle fibers to their final bony insertions are essential for optimal transmission of contractile forces.[55] They arise between the myofilaments to the endomysium and subsequent links to the perimysium, tendon, aponeuroses, and, finally, the bone. The muscle's capacity to transmit the contraction force can be impeded by damage or dysfunctional adaptive changes in any part of this link.[55–57]

Similar to connective tissue elsewhere, the muscles' fasciae and tendons adapt in response to changes in loading forces and patterns.[58] Relevant to exercise prescription is the adaptive restructuring observed during immobilization or restricted mobility. It manifests as an imbalance between the content of connective tissue and that of muscle fiber, decrease in the tissue's length, increased stiffness, and change in the overall architecture of the fascia.[55–57] Within 2 days of immobilization the ratio of collagen in muscle increases due to rapid atrophy of muscle fibers (in the shortened but not in the lengthened muscle).[55] Within 4 weeks of immobilization the muscle's fascia can shorten by as much as 25%.[59,60] Additionally, in immobilization the pennation angle of the muscle's fascicules tends to decrease, but it recovers rapidly following cast removal.[37,38,55] Notably, the dysfunctional effects of movement restriction can also be observed in the non-immobilized limb – a 15% decrease in connective tissue length and reorientation of the fibers.[59,60]

Generally, the morphological and biomechanical properties of muscle and the content of connective tissue tend to return to baseline within 8 weeks of remobilization.[37,38]

Clinical note: We can already see that muscles tend to adapt specifically to the person's principal physical activities. That is why the prescribed exercise has to closely resemble the activity which the individual aims to restore. This is the specificity principle in training. It has important implications for the physical form of the prescribed exercise (see Chapter 7). Maybe it is not a good idea to prescribe the injured marathon runner remedial weight training?

ADAPTATION IN THE NEUROLOGICAL DIMENSION: NEUROPLASTICITY

Our ability to learn a new skill, improve an existing one, or recover it after an injury or surgery is highly dependent on neuroplasticity – the adaptive

65. Hertz L, Chen Y. All 3 types of glial cells are important for memory formation. Front Integ Neurosci. 2016;10:31.

66. Elbert T, Pantev C, Wienbruch C, Rockstroh B, Taub E. Increased cortical representation of the fingers of the left hand in string players. Science. 1995;270:305–7.

67. Pascual-Leone A, Cohen LG, Hallett M. Cortical map plasticity in humans. Trends Neurosci. 1992;15:13–14.

68. Ungerleider LG, Doyon J, Karni A. Imaging brain plasticity during motor skill learning. Neurobiol Learn Mem. 2002;78:553–64.

69. Kidd G, Lawes N, Musa I. Understanding neuromuscular plasticity: a basis for clinical rehabilitation. Edward Arnold, London; 1992.

70. Rossi S, Pasqualetti P, Tecchio F, Sabato A, Rossini PM. Modulation of corticospinal output to human hand muscles following deprivation of sensory feedback. Neuroimage. 1998;8:163–75.

71. Seki K, Taniguchi Y, Narusawa M. Effects of joint immobilization on firing rate modulation of human motor units. J Physiol. 2001;530:507–19.

72. Karni A, Meyer G, Rey-Hipolito C, Jezzard P, Adams MM, Turner R, et al. The acquisition of skilled motor performance: fast and slow experience-driven changes in primary motor cortex. Proc Nat Acad Sci. 1998;95:861–8.

73. McComas AJ. Human neuromuscular adaptations that accompany changes in activity. Med Sci Sports Exerc. 1994;26:1498–1509.

74. Patten C, Kamen G. Adaptations in motor unit discharge activity with force control training in young and older human adults. Eur J Appl Physiol. 2000;83:128–43.

75. Duchateau J, Hainaut K. Effects of immobilization on contractile properties, recruitment and firing rates of human motor units. J Physiol. 1990;422:55–65.

76. de Jong BM, Coert JH, Stenekes MW, Leenders KL, Paans AM, Nicolai JP. Cerebral reorganisation of human hand movement following dynamic immobilisation. Neuroreport. 2003;14:1693–6.

77. Zanette G, Tinazzi M, Bonato C, di Summa A, Manganotti P, Polo A, et al. Reversible changes of motor cortical outputs following immobilization of the upper limb. Electroencephalogr Clin Neurophysiol. 1997;105: 269–79.

78. Cramer SC, Nelles G, Benson RR, Kaplan JD, Parker RA, Kwong KK, et al. A functional MRI study of subjects recovered from hemiparetic stroke. Stroke. 1997;28:2518–27.

79. Rowe JB, Frackowiak RS. The impact of brain imaging technology on our understanding of motor function and dysfunction. Curr Opin Neurobiol. 1999;9:728–34.

80. Jaalouk DE, Lammerding J. Mechanotransduction gone awry. Nat Rev Mol Cell Biol. 2009;10:63–73.

Chapter 7

Contents
The training conditions for functional adaptation

"You only learn, improve, or recover what you have practiced."

Imagine that you are prescribing exercise for a person following lower limb surgery, in which the goal of the management is to recover weight-bearing activities, such as walking. Ideally, the management should be efficient and effective, i.e., provide the minimum intervention to achieve maximum functionality, within the shortest time frame and with sustained long-term improvements. But how do we select the most effective management from the myriad of exercises recommended for leg rehabilitation? What would be better: practicing walking, or training using leg bench-presses or recumbent floor exercise? How similar to walking do the prescribed exercises have to be? Furthermore, how often and at what intensity should the exercise be practiced? Are there some universal principles for training that can direct us in planning a functional rehabilitation?

There are three key training principles from which a functional rehabilitation is constructed: *specificity*, *repetition*, and *intensity*.[1] Imagine that we have taken up a new skill: say, learning to play the piano. Instinctively, we would assume that practicing playing the banjo or exercising with a hand power grip is unlikely to support skillful piano playing. In order to learn or enhance this skill, we would have to practice playing the piano. In a similar way, rehabilitation of any task or activity is primarily influenced by practicing the task itself; hence, walking improves walking, a tennis serve is enhanced by practicing tennis serves, and so on. This principle is termed *training specificity*. Auxiliary exercises that are different from or dissimilar to the goal task are therefore unlikely to be as beneficial. So, training specificity can be summarized as: *practice what you aim to learn, improve, or recover.*

Repetition and frequent practice of the goal activity is another important principle in functional rehabilitation. We have the experience that the skillful or successful performance of a task is highly dependent on regular practice of that activity. Single episodes or long breaks in training are likely to result in poor performance, slow recovery, or even return of the adaptation to a disuse state, such as in detraining. In order to recover, say, walking after ankle immobilization, the patient will need numerous repetitions of dorsi-plantar flexion, with hundreds or even thousands of repetitions throughout the day, while sustaining this practice over several weeks or even months. Hence, the repetition principle can be summarized as: *practice what you aim to learn, improve, or recover – frequently.*

In some training programs the aim is to increase our physical capacity within the task, such as to lift heavier weights or run faster. This is often achieved by raising the physical or physiological demands during training above their present level. Hence, in order to run faster, we would increase the running speed during training, lift heavier weights to increase our capacity to lift, and so on. This training condition is often referred to as *training intensity*. This principle applies also to rehabilitation. For example, the weight-bearing capacity of the lower limb can be either attenuated by the use of crutches or progressively intensified by free walking, then walking faster, eventually moving on to use of stairs, and so on. In a nutshell, the three training conditions for adaptation can be summarized as: *only practice what you aim to recover or improve – frequently and (sometimes) more intensely.*

Chapter 7

THE SPECIFICITY CONDITION

When we learn a new skill, change the way we perform a task, or recover from an injury, our body undergoes a profound whole-person, multisystem adaptation. This adaptation is specific to that particular task.[2–8] It allows the task to be performed optimally with minimal expenditure of energy, physical stress, and error. Each task has its unique adaptive profile that is suitable for that activity but not exchangeable between dissimilar activities (Fig. 7.1).[9–11] This means that the remedial practice/training has to be similar,[12] if not identical, to the actual task/activity that we aim to recover: hence the terms *training specificity* or *task-specific rehabilitation*. If, for example, the goal is to rehabilitate a tennis serve or to walk, the training has to resemble these goal activities – ideally, using walking or tennis as the movement challenges. Auxiliary or extra-functional training, which is dissimilar to these activities, may be of little or no benefit for functional recovery. It raises the possibility that a wide array of commonly used auxiliary exercises will be of questionable remedial benefit to the person's functional repertoire, including weight training, resistance bands, stretching exercise, core and stabilization training, and so on.

Training specificity results in a unique adaptation that is observable from the molecular level, and in physiology and morphology, to the unique performance characteristic of the particular activity. For example, in muscle, specific adaptation is seen in response to endurance and resistance training. Differences can be seen in the expression of messenger RNA in the muscle's nuclei: 348 specific genes are expressed in resistance exercise and 48 genes in aerobic exercise.[13] Activity-specific adaptation can be seen in the capillary density, mitochondrial network, energy utilization, assembly of sarcomeres, fiber type, cross-section, length of muscle fascicle, and differences in the organization of sarcomeres.[14] Specificity does not end there. All these local changes are driven by the central nervous system (CNS) or the person. Unique task adaptation is also observed in CNS reorganization with changes in the sensorimotor areas of the brain and firing patterns of spinal motor neurons. Sprint and marathon running may look similar, yet each has its unique, non-transferable knee force-angle profile.[15] So, even the biomechanics are specific to the task. Hence, the specific structural, biomechanical, physiological, and neurological adaptation in one activity is unlikely to support the needs of another, dissimilar, one.

Specificity also implies – and this is very important – that there is no single universal exercise which can enhance the learning or performance of all human activities. This holy grail of rehabilitation and training has never been realized but is frequently promoted: for example, stretching exercise or strength training as the basis for remedial exercise. Each activity has its own unique adaptation. So, are there any training benefits that can be passed between two different activities?

Transfer of training

Imagine a clinical situation where a patient presents with difficulty in walking due to loss of force generation in the lower limb. Traditionally, to restore the power profile during walking, the patient is given a dissimilar auxiliary exercise: say, leg bench-presses. In prescribing the extra-functional exercises it is assumed that the force/power element within that activity would carry over to improve walking. This carry-over is called *transfer* – how the performance of a goal task (such as walking) is influenced by practice of another auxiliary activity (such as leg bench-presses).[10,16,17]

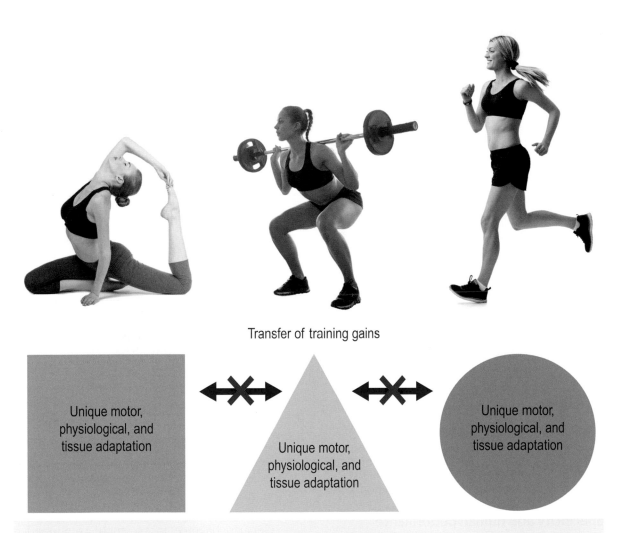

Transfer of training gains

Unique motor, physiological, and tissue adaptation

Unique motor, physiological, and tissue adaptation

Unique motor, physiological, and tissue adaptation

FIGURE 7.1

Training specificity. Tissue, motor, and physiological adaption is unique for each activity. Imagine you decide to take up a new activity such as yoga. Within a few months, your body will undergo dramatic adaptation, extending from the molecular–cellular level right up to the organs, and systemic to central nervous system. To some extent, after several months you will be a completely different person to when you started. If, after 6 months, you decide to switch to weight training, you will again undergo a total adaptive transformation to support the new activity. This whole-person metamorphosis will repeat itself if you decide after 6 months to switch to marathon running. *Importantly, the training gains from one activity will not carry over to support the next activity.* Nothing from the yoga training will help your weight training or running performance, and vice versa.

It is often believed that transfer can occur through particular components of movement. There are several movement components that are widely believed to be transferable:

- Task parameters: a common assumption is that transfer could be in one or several of the task parameters, such as force, velocity, range, and endurance (more in Chapter 8). It is often believed that training for endurance with leg-presses or cycling will improve endurance in standing and walking.

- Motor control components: there is a common belief that motor components, such as balance, coordination, and muscle recruitment sequences, are transferable between dissimilar tasks: for example, that trunk–pelvic–hip coordination and muscle recruitment timing during walking could be normalized by practicing these components on all fours or in a recumbent position. Similarly, people believe that the balance challenge of sitting on a Swiss ball would transfer to improvements in balance during walking.

So, how transferable are these movement components and what does the research demonstrate?

Specificity and human performance

Transfer has been studied extensively in the last few decades. Overall, these studies demonstrate that transfer of training gains rarely occurs between two dissimilar activities.[18] This phenomenon can already be observed in young children.[5] Each task in their movement repertoire is learned specifically, with little or no transfer between tasks, even those that share the same motor components. For example, a high level of fine hand coordination in drawing does not transfer to handling Lego bricks, and vice versa.

- **Transfer of strength, endurance, and velocity:** different forms of resistance exercise have failed to enhance sports-specific activities such as soccer kicks, sprinting, netball, hockey, throwing velocity in water polo, and rowing.[19-25] As for velocity, it seems that the intention to move faster is the key to improving speed of movement in sports;[26] for endurance, trunk endurance training may positively affect trunk muscle recruitment in this particular activity but it does not transfer to improvements in functional tasks or running economy.[27,28] There is also a possibility for negative transfer where the auxiliary activity interferes with the goal task: for example, cross-training in cycling does not improve running economy and may even reduce it.[29]

- **Mismatch in transfer goals:** often, transfer fails when there is a mismatch between the components challenged in the auxiliary exercise and those targeted in the goal activity. For example, training in isolated tasks, such as hip flexibility or trunk-strengthening activities, does not improve the economy of walking or running.[30]

- **Balance and coordination transfer:** auxiliary training in balance can improve performance in this activity but may have only minor or no transfer to the goal task.[31-34] Generic balance tasks, such as a one-leg stance, may have little value as an overall balance measure. In elite gymnasts or athletes (judo and dance), training to perform difficult, sport-specific postures does not transfer balance ability to commonly used standing postures.[35-38] Core stability training, focused on abdominal muscle control and coordination, fails to improve sports performance.[39-43] Unfortunately, challenging coordination in salsa dancing fails to improve the performance of cross-country skiing (yes, someone has tried that).[44]

- **Transfer between similar tasks:** transfer may fail, even in types of auxiliary training that seem to closely resemble the goal task. For example, resistance training in one particular posture may not transfer strength gains to other postures.[35–38,45] Resistance sprint training using a weighted towing device fails to improve sprint performance.[46] Similarly, off-ice "dry" skating exercises do not improve on-ice performance in speed skaters.[47] Vertical jumps are improved by training in vertical jumps but not by training in sideways jumps.[48] Sprinting performance was shown to improve by practicing single-leg horizontal jumps but not vertical jumps using both limbs, such as jump squats.[22] Even what seem like minor changes in the goal task may not transfer well. For example, strength gains are greatest at the training velocity and movement range, with only some carry-over to other velocities and angles.[49–54] Yes, specificity can be that finicky. It means that if the aim is to increase speed performance – say, in tennis or walking – lifting heavy weights at low velocity might be counterproductive.

There is also the potential issue of negative transfer, where the auxiliary training may interfere with the performance of the goal activity. For example, eccentric cycling induces muscle hypertrophy and augments eccentric strength.[55] These gains do not transfer into improvements in cycling performance and, conversely, seem to have a limiting or detrimental effect on this skill.

There is also a clinical illusion of transfer (Fig. 7.2). Imagine a situation where a soccer player is prescribed auxiliary strengthening exercise. In subsequent clinical sessions, they demonstrate a substantial improvement in that activity. However, within the clinical setup we have no means to track their improvement in soccer. Consequently, on the basis of our clinical findings, we may come to the wrong assumption that their soccer performance has benefited too. Another illusion of transfer is when a skilled individual switches from their principal sport to another similar one: say, from badminton to tennis. Interestingly, they will still have to undergo sports-specific adaptation. So, for several months they tend to play "tenniston," using badminton movement patterns to play tennis. It will take them about 6 months to establish a true tennis-playing style.

Overall, in order to enhance task performance, the training should closely resemble the goal task. But what about individuals who are recovering from a musculoskeletal condition? Does the specificity principle still apply?

Specificity reasoning:

Q: What would be the best training to learn or improve, say, a tennis serve [or insert here any other activity]?

A: Most people would correctly answer – practice playing tennis.

Q: What about the "second-best" training for tennis: what would that look like?

A: Different answers are possible, depending on who is asked. Often suggested is upper limb resistance training, stretching, and so on; occasionally, the answer remains unchanged – play tennis – which is the correct response.

Q: Let's assume, for the sake of debate, that a second-best training is useful. Then the question is, why would we ever choose the second best if we can train in the best?

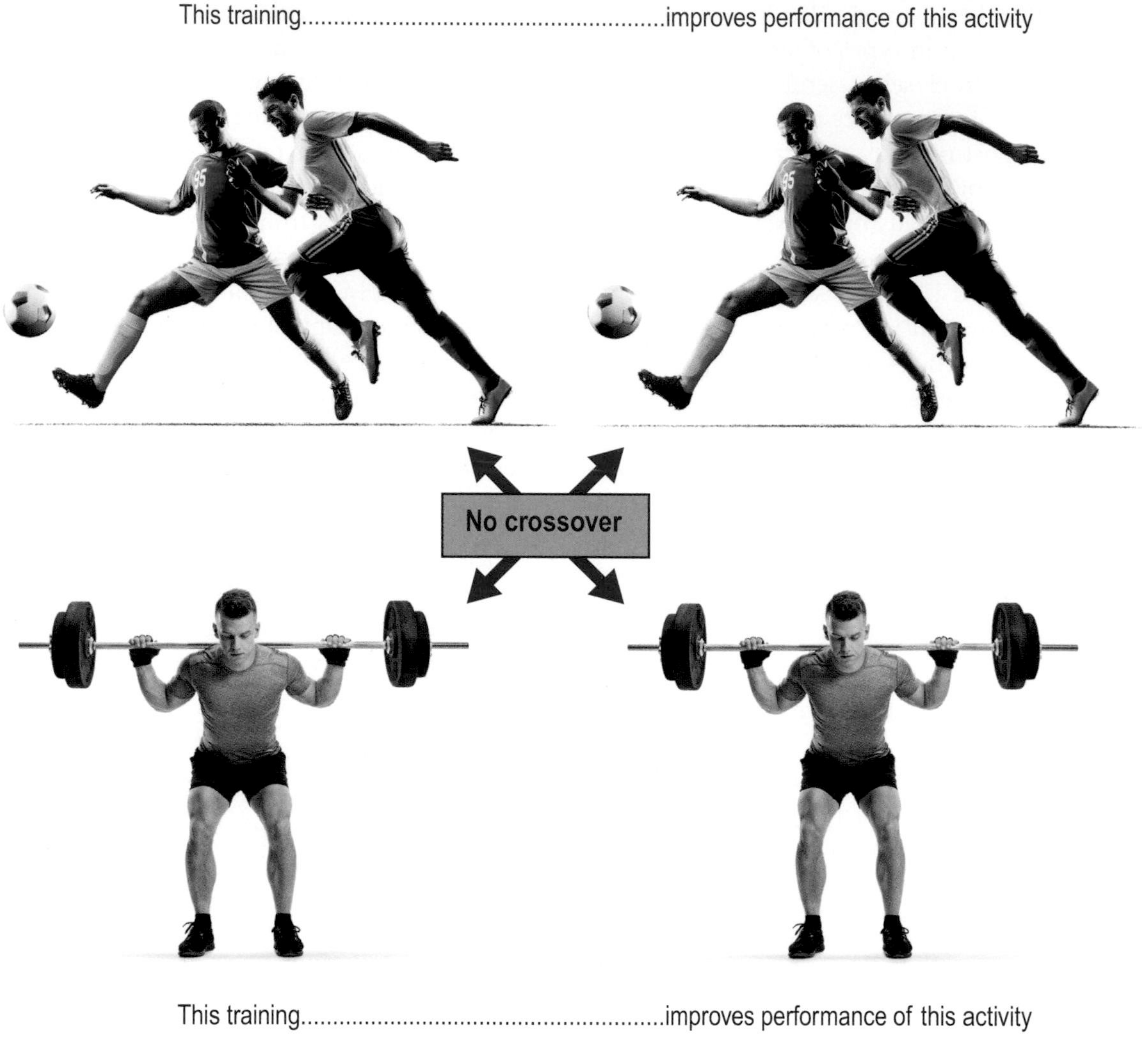

This training...improves performance of this activity

No crossover

This training...improves performance of this activity

FIGURE 7.2
The clinical illusion of transfer. Clinical improvements in auxiliary training do not represent improvements in the goal activity.

Specificity in movement rehabilitation

The phenomenon of specificity and transfer has largely focused on neurorehabilitation but is otherwise neglected in post-injury/surgery management.[1]

In individuals suffering from chronic neck pain, extra-functional neck exercises (resistance and endurance) do not transfer to improvement in functional head–neck movements.[56] A positive transfer of postural stability was demonstrated in a study of balance in subjects with lateral ankle sprain. In laboratory studies, training under moderately unstable conditions transferred to improvements in postural control under more challenging stability conditions.[57] However, these improvements may not transfer to functional activities outside the laboratory. For example, balance training on a wobble board does not reduce the incidence of ankle sprains which may be associated with lower limb coordination deficits.[58] A recent systematic review suggests that, in the elderly, the transfer of physical benefits from resistance strength training to activities of daily living performance, such as walking, seems to be limited.[59] In a small study on elderly individuals, it was found that training in functional activities gave the same strength gains in the legs as exercising using resistance bands.[60] However, the functional training also conferred greater improvements in dynamic balance control and coordination while performing daily life tasks. In a similar but larger study, functional exercises were found to be more effective than resistance exercises at improving functional task performance in healthy elderly women.[61]

Studies of individuals with age-related or pathological ROM losses suggest a lack of transfer between auxiliary stretching exercise and improvement in functional movement ranges. A study of older women found no effect of regular exercise and stretching on walking performance.[62] Similarly, in a study of older individuals with hip flexor contracture, 8 weeks of hip and ankle stretching provided a modestly improved passive ROM (hip 6.8°, ankle 3.5°) but failed to improve stride length.[63] In a similar study, 10 weeks of hip and ankle stretching improved hip flexibility (1.5°) but failed to show significant improvements in gait performance. Twelve weeks of foot exercise that included ankle stretching failed to improve functional gait performance in elderly individuals.[64] A Cochrane systematic review reported that various forms of traditional stretching exercise for contractures failed to improve functional activities (but that could be also associated with the ineffectiveness of stretching to improve tissue extensibility).[65]

In stroke patients, resistance cycling or seated strength exercise improves strength in these activities but has little or no effect on walking.[66,67] Similarly, sitting and reaching training improves sitting and reaching and the production of vertical force through the leg as they lean forward.[68] The vertical force improvement in the leg seems to transfer to an improvement in getting up from sitting, but nothing from that training transfers to walking. However, training of stroke patients in walking improves walking speed and distance but not balance.[69–71] Balance seems to be improved by challenging balance.[72,73] Nevertheless, challenging static balance in standing might not transfer well to dynamic balance during walking.[74] So, here too, transfer can be unpredictable and finicky. This specificity message has been stated in a recent systematic review of stroke rehabilitation: there is strong evidence for physical therapy interventions favoring intensive highly repetitive task-oriented and task-specific training in all phases post-stroke. Importantly, the effects were found to be restricted to the functions and activities actually trained for.[75]

Overall, several decades of research suggest that specificity is the dominant outcome of training/practice and that transfer between dissimilar tasks is unpredictable, mostly absent, and if present, is considered to be modest: i.e., we cannot foresee which auxiliary training will benefit the activity that we are trying to improve.[76,77] Perhaps the time has come to eliminate management that relies on auxiliary exercise and transfer. But how?

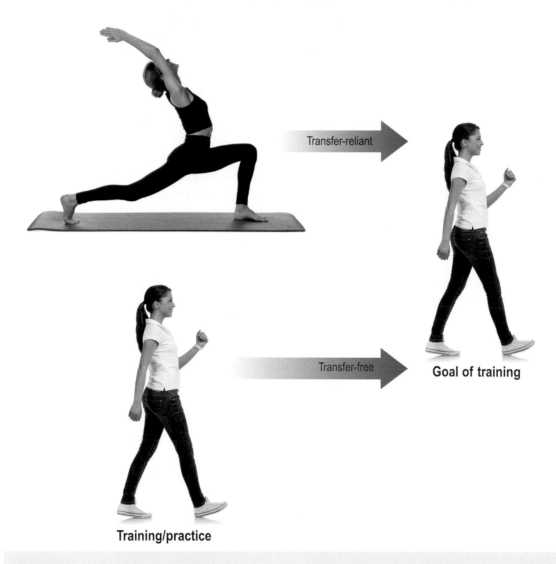

Transfer-reliant

Transfer-free

Goal of training

Training/practice

FIGURE 7.3
The reliance on transfer of training gains can be abolished by practicing the goal activity.

Eliminating transfer

If we browse through any rehabilitation publication or website, the majority of exercises prescribed are likely to be auxiliary in form, with little or no resemblance to the way humans move in their daily or sports activities.[78] There is a misguided belief that the more outlandish the exercise is, the more therapeutic value it has.

Yet, the likelihood for transfer diminishes as the dissimilarity between the auxiliary and the goal activity widens. The simple solution is to eliminate the dependency on transfer by minimizing the use of auxiliary exercise – basically, by practicing the goal tasks as closely as possible to their functional manifestation (Fig. 7.3). This can reduce the ineffectiveness and unpredictability that are inherent in transfer from the auxiliary training. For example, a patient who is unable to get up from sitting due to a lower limb condition is often prescribed exercise such as half-squats leaning against a wall, or seated resisted knee extensions, and so on. These exercises are too dissimilar to the actual activity and rely heavily on transfer. The simple alternative is just to practice sit-to-stand from a raised seat. This task variation is similar and transfer-free.

Generalization of task

We all have the experience in which we need to modify a habitual daily task without a protracted learning phase, such as driving an unfamiliar hired car without having to relearn driving. If specificity in adaptation was absolute, it would mean that we would have to learn the task, including each of its infinite variations. This problem in adaptation is overcome by our ability to extend our learning or training experiences to variations of *the same* activity or task. This ability is called task *generalization*.[79–82]

When novices learn a new activity, they often add an element of variability into the practice, such as taking basketball shots from different positions. In reality, we never repeat a movement in exactly the same manner. As Heraclitus of Ephesus (475 BCE) stated: "No man ever steps in the same river twice," or as one of his students remarked, "No SAME man ever steps in the same river twice." Hence, every step we make and every breath we take and every tennis serve

we perform will be different from any other. The vast constellation of factors in each iteration is never the same (although they may look as if they are). So, task variability is naturally present during all learning and training. Later, variability provides us with some generalization capacity.[83] It enables us to modify the task in the future without having to learn each variation from scratch or practice the task in all its infinite versions.[84–86] Hence, a skillful basketball shot can be performed in situations that have never been encountered during training,[87] to which Heraclitus would have remarked that no same man takes the same basketball shot twice.

In summary, the message to exercise prescription from science is clear. You can vary the task but do not expect transfer between dissimilar tasks. A person can be instructed to walk with a wider stride (generalization) but do not expect transfer between, say, core stability training and walking.

The home laboratory: experience generalization by holding a pen between the thumb and the last three fingers rather than the usual thumb and index finger. Try to write. You are likely to find it fairly easy, although you have never written using this unusual pen hold.

Some thoughts on specificity of training:

"You only learn what you have practiced (you can't learn what you haven't practiced)."

"You only adapt to what you have practiced (you can't adapt to what you haven't practiced)."

"Practice what you aim to recover (and the body will follow)."

"(Specific) practice makes perfect."

REPETITION CONDITION

Repeated practice is an important driver for learning a new skill, enhancing current skills, and supporting long-term improvements in functional recovery.[75,76,88] Recurrent exposure to an activity is associated with extensive molecular reprogramming within the nervous system and musculoskeletal system that leads to long-term adaptation.[89,90] But what is the optimal practice schedule to drive these long-term adaptations?

Scheduling of prescribed exercise is a common clinical conundrum. "How long for and how often" is one of the first questions asked when constructing the exercise management. The answer is not straightforward. The scheduling advice depends on a multitude of factors, such as the complexity of the goal task, extent of pathology, tissues affected, length of detraining period, age, other medical conditions, and time available to practice, to name but a few.

The duration component of scheduling can be informed by looking at what level of activity maintains our natural functional capacity. Essentially, our capacity to carry out daily activities is maintained by the duration of and repeated engagement in these activities – the numerous steps or the frequent reaching and retrieving actions we perform throughout the day. We do not need to increase the time spent on these familiar activities in order to preserve them. So, the pre-injury functional capacity becomes the rehabilitation target. Imagine a person with a leg injury who could walk 1 hour in the past but now can manage only 15 minutes. These post- and pre-injury durations can become the management parameters: increase walking duration from 15 minutes to 1 hour. Similarly, with an injured runner, the management goal would be to increase their post-injury capacity of, say, 10 minutes back to the pre-injury level of 1.5 hours. In the ideal recovery scenario, once these remedial targets are met, the improvements are sustained by the individual's engagement in these specific activities. So, now we have the start and end duration in any particular activity.

The post- to pre-injury activity duration can be managed by using activity grading (see Chapter 9). The activity's duration can be increased incrementally week by week. There is no strict rule about the size of the increment, except that it has to be realistic, effective, and memorable for the patient. The schedule could start as a daily engagement in the particular activity, within the individual's current capacity: say, 5 minutes' walk. This duration can be increased incrementally week by week, for example by 10% or 20%, until the individual achieves their 100% – or near enough – goal duration in the affected activity. If necessary, the duration of the daily exposure can be broken into smaller units, e.g., three 10-minute walks rather than a single 30-minute spell. Basically, the scheduling is tweaked as you go along.

In a functional approach, there is no clear boundary between "exercising" and engaging in activities of daily living: i.e., the shared repertoire. So, another, less structured scheduling approach is to encourage the individual to engage in the affected activities as often as possible. A person with limited shoulder range can be encouraged to favor the affected arm in reaching and retrieving activities and to swing it a bit further when walking (see Chapter 14 for examples). These and other arm-related activities can be repeated, as often as possible, throughout the day. This simple management could chalk up a substantial daily repetition of shoulder challenges.

Scheduling for skill learning and enhancing performance

Exercise prescription is often about improving or correcting the performance of a pre-existing activity. The focus here is on the skill proficiency or the performance style – more about "how well" than "how much." There is a wide spectrum of conditions which are covered by this form of management, such as advice about posture, and bending and lifting techniques. It also relates to instructions about modifying incorrect or ineffective movement in sports activities, such as advice about landing techniques in volleyball to prevent lower limb injuries, or enhancing swimming performance by modifying the stroke style. Performance and skill enhancement are largely dependent on motor learning processes, which determine the practice schedule.

There are two motor control issues to consider in performance and skill enhancement: learning a new task and enhancing the performance of a familiar pre-existing skill; for example, the difference between learning a tennis serve from scratch versus improving an existing serving skill. There are dramatic scheduling differences between the two learning scenarios. Many daily activities which we perform without a thought were acquired and refined over several years and numerous repetitions. For example, learning to walk evolves over 6–10 years with several million step repetitions. Mastering accuracy in basketball requires some 1 million baskets shots. On the other hand, learning a minor variation of an existing skill may take a few attempts and may be polished within days or a few weeks. To learn a modified landing technique, experienced athletes may require as few as 20 repetitions or three weekly training sessions over 6 weeks to acquire the skill and retain it for up to a year.[91,92] Note that these studies were conducted in a movement laboratory setting; we do not know if learning of the modified landing technique would transfer to a real-world situation during a game.

"Practice what you aim to recover – frequently."

INTENSITY OF TRAINING

The intensity of the training condition is mostly about "how much" rather than "how well." Losses in capacity are often seen in injury, immobilization, and detraining situations, and tend to affect any of the four movement parameters – force, endurance, range, and velocity (see Chapter 8). These movement parameters can be the target of exercise prescription and their intensity can be either amplified or attenuated, depending on the patient's condition. Take a daily activity such as walking: within this activity, the intensity of these four parameters can be modified without changing walking itself. We can increase the force component by walking up a hill or stairs, or simply by stepping up the pace of walking (force and velocity). The duration of walking can be extended (endurance), as well as the stride length (range). But how do we know by how much?

As with the scheduling principle described above, the limits of intensity are defined by the individual's pre- and post-injury capacity levels. The individual's pre-injury functional capacity is the goal and the post-injury deficits represent the rehabilitation starting point. For example, for a person who had leg surgery, recovering sit-to-stand ability can start from a comfortable and achievable seat height (e.g., raised with cushions) and be lowered incrementally until the functional level is restored (see Chapter 14 for a demonstration). Similarly, the speed capacity of a runner can be incrementally increased from the post- to the pre-injury levels, and so on. These principles are discussed in greater detail in Chapters 8 and 9.

28. Tse MA, McManus AM, Masters RS. Development and validation of a core endurance intervention program: implications for performance in college-age rowers. J Strength Cond Res. 2005;19:547–52.

29. Pizza FX, Flynn MG, Starling RD, Brolinson PG, Sigg J, Kubitz ER, et al. Run training vs cross training: influence of increased training on running economy, foot impact shock and run performance. Int J Sports Med. 1995;16:180–4.

30. Godges JJ, MacRae PG, Engelke KA. Effects of exercise on hip range of motion, trunk muscle performance, and gait economy. Phys Ther. 1993;73:468–77.

31. Casabona A, Leonardi G, Aimola E, La Grua G, Polizzi CM, Cioni M, et al. Specificity of foot configuration during bipedal stance in ballet dancers. Gait Posture. 2016;46:91–7.

32. Giboin LS, Gruber M, Kramer A. Task-specificity of balance training. Hum Mov Sci. 2015;44:22–31.

33. Donath L, Roth R, Zahner L, Faude O. Slackline training (balancing over narrow nylon ribbons) and balance performance: a meta-analytical review. Sports Med. 2017;47:1075–86.

34. Kümmel J, Kramer A, Giboin LS, Gruber M. Specificity of balance training in healthy individuals: a systematic review and meta-analysis. Sports Med. 2016;46:1261–71.

35. Aseman F, Caron O, Cremieux J. Is there a transfer of postural ability from specific to unspecific postures in elite gymnasts? Neurosci Lett. 2004;358:83–6.

36. Paillard T, Noe F, Riviere T. Performance and strategy in the unipedal stance of soccer players at different levels of competition. J Athl Train. 2006;41:172–6.

37. Paillard T, Costes-Salon MC, Lafont C, Dupui P. Are there differences in postural regulation according to the level of competition in judoists? Br J Sports Med. 2002;36:304–5.

38. Simmons RW. Sensory organization determinants of postural stability in trained ballet dancers. Int J Neuro. 2005;115:87–97.

39. Hibbs AE, Thompson KG, French D, Wrigley A, Spears I. Optimizing performance by improving core stability and core strength. Sports Med. 2008;38:995–1008.

40. Reed CA, Ford KR, Myer GD, Hewett TE. The effects of isolated and integrated 'core stability' training on athletic performance measures: a systematic review. Sports Med. 2012;42:697–706.

41. Wirth K, Hartmann H, Mickel C, Szilas E, Keiner M, Sander A. Core stability in athletes: a critical analysis of current guidelines. Sports Med. 2017;47:401–14.

42. Parkhouse KL, Ball N. Influence of dynamic versus static core exercises on performance in field based fitness tests. J Bodyw Mov Ther. 2011;15:517–24.

43. Okada T, Huxel KC, Nesser TW. Relationship between core stability, functional movement, and performance. J Strength Cond Res. 2011;25:252–61.

44. Alricsson M, Werner S. The effect of pre-season dance training on physical indices and back pain in elite cross-country skiers: a prospective controlled intervention study. Br J Sports Med. 2004;38:148–53.

45. Wilson GJ, Murphy AJ, Walshe A. The specificity of strength training: the effect of posture. Eur J Appl Physiol Occup Physiol. 1996;73:346–52.

46. Kristensen GO, van den Tillaar R, Ettema GJ. Velocity specificity in early-phase sprint training. J Strength Cond Res. 2006;20:833–7.

47. de Boer RW, Ettema GJ, Faessen BG, Krekels H, Hollander AP, de Groot G, et al. Specific characteristics of speed skating: implications for summer training. Med Sci Sports Exerc. 1987;19:504–10.

48. King JA, Cipriani DJ. Comparing preseason frontal and sagittal plane plyometric programs on vertical jump height in high-school basketball players. J Strength Cond Res. 2010;24:2109–14.

49. Folland JP, Hawker K, Leach B, Little T, Jones DA. Strength training: isometric training at a range of joint angles versus dynamic training. J Sports Sci. 2005;23:817–24.

50. Weir JP, Housh DJ, Housh TJ, Weir LL. The effect of unilateral eccentric weight training and detraining on joint angle specificity, cross-training, and the bilateral task deficit. J Orthop Sports Phys Ther. 1995;22:207–15.

51. Morrissey MC, Harman EA, Johnson MJ. Resistance training modes: specificity and effectiveness. Med Sci Sports Exerc. 1995;27:648–60.

52. Ingebrigtsen J, Holtermann A, Roeleveld K. Effects of load and contraction velocity during three-week biceps curls training on isometric and isokinetic performance. J Strength Cond Res. 2009;23:1670–6.

53. Blazevich AJ, Jenkins D. Physical performance differences between weight-trained sprinters and weight trainers. J Sci Med Sport. 1998;1:12–21.

54. Pereira MIR, Gomes PSC. Movement velocity in resistance training. Sports Med. 2003;33:427–38.

55. Paulsen G, Eidsheim HØ, Helland C, Seynnes O, Solberg PA, Rønnestad BR. Eccentric cycling does not improve cycling performance in amateur cyclists. PLoS One. 2019;14:e0208452.

56. Falla D, Jull G, Hodges P. Training the cervical muscles with prescribed motor tasks does not change muscle activation during a functional activity. Man Ther. 2008;13:507–12.

57. Rotem-Lehrer N, Laufer Y. Effect of focus of attention on transfer of a postural control task following an ankle sprain. J Orthop Sports Phys Ther. 2007;37:564–9.

58. Postle K, Pak D, Smith TO. Effectiveness of proprioceptive exercises for ankle ligament injury in adults: a systematic literature and meta-analysis. Man Ther. 2012;17:285–91.

59. Liu C-J, Shiroy DM, Jones LY, Clark DO. Systematic review of functional training on muscle strength, physical functioning, and activities of daily living in older adults. Eur Rev Aging Phys Activ. 2014;11:144.

60. Krebs D, Scarborough DM, McGibbon CA. Functional vs. strength training in disabled elderly outpatients. Am J Phys Med Rehab. 2007;86:93–103.

61. de Vreede PL, Samson MM, van Meeteren NL, Duursma SA, Verhaar HJ. Functional-task exercise versus resistance strength exercise to improve daily function in older women: a randomized, controlled trial. J Am Geriatr Soc. 2005;53:2–10.

62. Reis JG, Costa GC, Schmidt A, Ferreira CH, Abreu DC. Do muscle strengthening exercises improve performance in the 6-minute walk test in post-menopausal women? Braz J PhysTher. 2012;16:236–40.

63. Christiansen CL. The effects of hip and ankle stretching on gait function of older people. Arch Phys Med Rehabil. 2008; 89:1421–8.

64. Hartmann A, Murer K, de Bie RA, de Bruin ED. The effect of a foot gymnastic exercise programme on gait performance in older adults: a randomised controlled trial. Disabil Rehabil. 2009;31:2101–10.

65. Harvey LA, Katalinic OM, Herbert RD, Moseley AM, Lannin NA, Schurr K. Stretch for the treatment and prevention of contractures. Cochrane Database Syst Rev. 2017 Jan 9;1:CD007455.

66. Sullivan KJ, Brown DA, Klassen T, Mulroy S, Ge T, Azen SP, et al. Effects of task-specific locomotor and strength training in adults who were ambulatory after stroke: results of the STEPS randomized clinical trial. Phys Ther. 2007;87:1580–602; discussion 1603–7.

67. Flansbjer UB, Miller M, Downham D, Lexell J. Progressive resistance training after stroke: effects on muscle strength, muscle tone, gait performance and perceived participation. J Rehabil Med. 2008;40:42–8.

68. Dean CM, Channon EF, Hall JM. Sitting training early after stroke improves sitting ability and quality and carries over to standing up but not to walking: a randomised trial. Aust J Physiother. 2007;53:97–102.

69. van de Port IG, Wood-Dauphinee S, Lindeman E, Kwakkel G. Effects of exercise training programs on walking competency after stroke: a systematic review. Am J Phys Med Rehabil. 2007;86:935 51.

70. Van Peppen RP, Kwakkel G, Wood-Dauphinee W, Hendriks HJM, Van der Wees PhH, Dekker J. The impact of physical therapy on functional outcomes after stroke: what's the evidence? Clin Rehabil. 2004;18:833–62.

71. Bogey R, Hornby GT. Gait training strategies utilized in poststroke rehabilitation: are we really making a difference? Top Stroke Rehabil. 2007;14:1–8.

72. de Haart M, Geurts AC, Huidekoper SC, Fasotti L, van Limbeek J. Recovery of standing balance in postacute stroke patients: a rehabilitation cohort study. Arch Phys Med Rehabil. 2004;85:886–95.

73. Sherrington C, Whitney JC, Lord SR, Herbert RD, Cumming RG, Close JCT. Effective exercise for the prevention of falls: a systematic review and meta-analysis. J Am Geriatr Soc. 2008;56:2234–43.

Chapter 8

Contents
Exercise prescription: task, component, and movement focus

Imagine a situation where gait is rehabilitated after a lower limb condition, particularly in the latter phase of repair. The person's condition has shifted from an inflammatory phase and a proliferating phase towards a remodeling phase. Their tissues are rapidly restoring their biomechanical properties, symptoms subside, and the patient is instinctively drawn to resume functional activities. At this juncture, where is the focus and what is the aim of rehabilitation?

There are several management choices here. One approach could be just to practice the whole task, e.g., use walking to rehabilitate walking – referred to as *task-focused rehabilitation*. Another focus could be on particular elements of walking, such as balance, force, endurance, and so on – referred to as *component-focused rehabilitation*. Or management could

focus on correcting or modifying the walking movement patterns – termed *movement-focused rehabilitation* (Fig. 8.1A–C).

So, how do we go about deciding which level to focus on?

TASK-FOCUSED REHABILITATION

"Focus on the task and let the body organize the rest."

Task-focused management is about the skillful performance of an activity. In task-focused rehabilitation, the patient is encouraged to practice the affected task as a whole, within the constraints of their condition. A person walking with a limp due to a lower limb condition could be advised to walk, even with a limp. A person suffering from chronic back pain with limited trunk movement could be advised

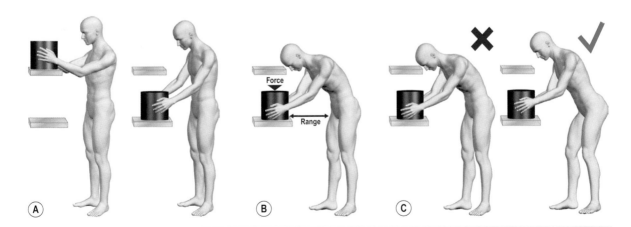

FIGURE 8.1
Focus of rehabilitation. (A) Task-focused rehabilitation: practicing the whole task. (B) Task component focus: same task but modifying the range and force component. (C) Movement-focused rehabilitation: same task but modifying the movement associated with the task ("correctness of movement").

to keep on trying to bend, twist, and lift. Task-focused rehabilitation is also used to enhance and recover skillful performance of activities, in situations such as those that follow long-term disuse or detraining. This approach is also used in central nervous system (CNS) conditions: for example, retraining a stroke patient to reuse their hand in daily activities, such as the skillful use of a fork, lifting a cup, and so on. It is expected that, in time, the activities in focus will "normalize" through repeated daily use. This, by the way, is how most individuals recover from the multitude of injuries they suffer throughout life.

So, what is the reasoning for choosing task-focused management and what happens if we stray from this approach? In order to answer these questions, we need to explore the role of motor control in functional rehabilitation and, in particular, how movement is organized as goal and whole.

Goal-oriented movement

We all have had the experience of practicing a new activity; after a while, we do not have to think about how to carry it out and it seems to occur just by "willing" it. This is a motor learning phenomenon associated with a transition in skill acquisition from a *cognitive* to a subconscious *autonomous* phase: a sort of "beginner" to "expert" state (Fig. 8.2).[1]

The early cognitive stages of learning are characterized by a high level of conscious activity focused on the task's particulars and its related movement. As the individual becomes more proficient in performing a skill, it becomes more autonomous and less under conscious control. At this stage, the task and the related movement are integrated centrally and executed

as a whole.[2–4] This integration is so smooth that, throughout the day, we carry out numerous activities while being completely oblivious to the movement that supports them. If you were instructed to touch your phone (if you do not mind just doing that), you will realize that it just happens. You did not have to consider the position of your arm, the elbow angle, the force generated by the biceps, and so on. Our movements are organized around goals or a purpose – we reach for a cup, hit a ball, walk to a location – but we do not set out to move our limbs, move a joint, or contract a muscle.[5,6] At the autonomous phase, the movement and the task/goal are seamlessly and robustly integrated, and consequently, it is difficult to remodel the movement patterns of long-standing, well-rehearsed habits: for example, an experienced sports person learning a new tennis serve or swimming stroke.

Another feature of the transition from the cognitive to the autonomous phase is in the focus of attention.[7] When we focus on the workings of our body and the task-related movement, it is referred to as an *internal focus of attention*. This form of attention is associated with the early cognitive learning phase. Once a person becomes skilled, their attention is directed toward the goal of the activity (grab the phone) – termed the *external focus of attention* (Fig. 8.2). Both internal and external focuses of attention have their place in motor learning. When learning an activity from scratch – e.g., a tennis serve – it initially requires an internal focus of attention.[8] At this stage, the person is learning the basic principles of the task, how to hold the racket, how to serve, how to stand, and a host of other aspects of the movement. Once they acquire the basic principles of the movement, they tend to shift towards an external focus of attention, such as landing the

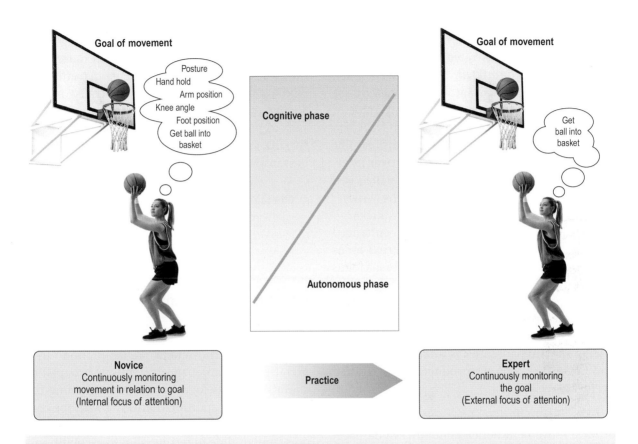

FIGURE 8.2
During motor learning, there is a transition from the cognitive–novice to an autonomous–expert phase. In the early phase, the individual is internally focused on their body, its position, and the principles of the task in relation to the goal. In the autonomous phase, the body "vanishes" as the individual becomes externally focused on the goal.

ball on a specific part of their opponent's court.[9] At that point, the individual becomes "oblivious" to the workings of their body.

The shift from internal to external focus is universal to all skill-learning processes. However – importantly – it does not work in reverse. When an expert is instructed to focus internally and re-examine their movement, their performance tends to degrade in terms of learning, accuracy, and movement economy. In a study of basketball free throws, participants were given internal focus (wrist motion) and external focus (basket) instructions.[10] During the throws, electromyography (EMG) activity was recorded in the participants' shooting arm. Throws performed with an external focus resulted in greater accuracy and lower

EMG activity, indicating an enhanced economy of movement. This advantage in movement economy was demonstrated even in the simple task of lifting a dumbbell. Subjects were given the instruction to focus either externally on the goal height or internally on the elbow angle or biceps activity.[11,12] Again, lower EMG activity was seen in the external focus condition. The performance advantages of external over internal focus have been shown in sports such as golf (focus on the goal versus focus on the wrist),[13] serves in volleyball, and soccer kicks.[14,15] Similarly, balance performance is enhanced with an external rather than an internal focus (e.g., focus on a spot in the distance versus focus on your feet).[16] Even conscious tensing of the trunk muscles (internal focus) has been shown to degrade postural control.[17] So, advising people to focus internally and "engage their core" during sporting activities is totally unnecessary and probably counterproductive to skilled performance.[18]

Individuals who have been injured, are in pain, or have movement deficits due to CNS damage, tend naturally to focus on their body, which may further degrade their movement performance.[19] This effect was demonstrated in baseball position players who recovered from knee surgery and pitchers who recovered from elbow surgery, up to 18 months post-surgery.[19] The position players had an internal focus of attention localized to the knee, whereas the injured pitchers had a diffuse, internal focus. In both groups, the internal focus was associated with inferior performance relative to non-injured athletes. It implies that, following injury, movement recovery can be enhanced by trainings which emphasize an external focus of attention. For example, a person recovering from elbow surgery can be given graded arm-reaching activities

with external focus instructions such as "reach for the water bottle," rather than focusing internally on strengthening specific arm muscles or the position of the limb. The beneficial effects of external focus have been demonstrated in balancing and walking performance in conditions such as postural steadiness deficits due to ankle sprains, and CNS conditions such as stroke and Parkinson's disease.[20–23]

> **Message to the patient:** "keep your eyes on the goal, not on your body." Try to steer the person away from training trends which overfocus on the body.

Whole versus fragmentation

"Integrate in order to coordinate."

Traditionally, movement rehabilitation uses exercises that target specific muscle group(s) or chain(s), such as focusing on strengthening the quads in knee conditions, working with the core muscles for back pain sufferers, or concentrating on scapular glide to resolve shoulder conditions. These practices follow the traditional training maxim *"fragment in order to integrate."* Although movement fragmentation is widely used in all forms of exercise therapy and training, is it beneficial?

Movement fragmentation can be explored by looking at the extent of muscle recruitment during movement. When we perform any activity, our whole body is organized for it, head to toe. One way to visualize the motor output is to imagine a person wearing a full body-suit covered with LED lights that represent the activity intensity of the underlying muscles. If this was possible, we would probably see a psychedelic whole-body light show, continuously changing as the person moves or even while they are being still.[24] Some areas will show low or even silent phases of inactivity (called surround inhibition) in both static and dynamic activities.[25,26] These relaxed muscle groups are also part of the movement plan. Without their silence, that task cannot be accomplished, e.g., relaxation of the back muscles during forward bending.[27] From a motor control perspective, movement is organized as a whole – there is no single, group-specific, or subsystem muscle recruitment (Fig. 8.3A&B).

The motor system does not have a recruitment hierarchy: no muscle is more important than another, and they are all organized to support the task optimally. Importantly, it is the task which determines the muscles' recruitment

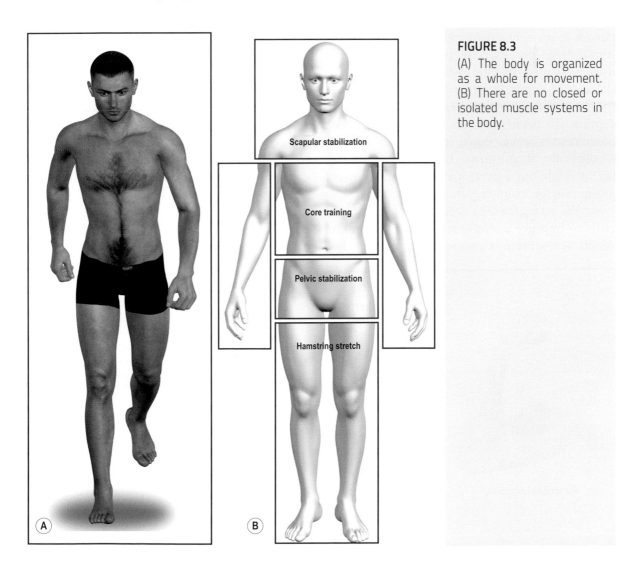

Scapular stabilization

Core training

Pelvic stabilization

Hamstring stretch

(A)

(B)

FIGURE 8.3
(A) The body is organized as a whole for movement. (B) There are no closed or isolated muscle systems in the body.

pattern (Fig. 8.4).[28–30] So, the same muscle will have different recruitment patterns, depending on the task (Fig. 8.5). All the hand muscles participate in writing, knitting, or rolling dough, but none of these muscles is specific to any of these particular activities. Equally, there are no specific stabilizers, prime movers, or postural muscles.[31,32] From a motor system perspective, the task determines the muscle recruitment.

Task-determined recruitment and whole-person movement organization have important implications for exercise prescription. Often, muscle- or joint-specific exercises are given with the aim of improving the whole task. However, this kind of fragmentation is a training misconception. To begin with, no matter how far the movement is broken down, it will always involve whole-body recruitment. It is near impossible to single out a particular muscle or muscle group. So, for example, what happens when we prescribe strengthening exercise such as biceps curls to improve a tennis serve? Ask the brain. As far as the brain is concerned, its master, the

person, is ordering it to learn a new activity called biceps curls – a new task, with a new title and completely new whole-body muscle recruitment. However, these recruitment patterns will be great for biceps curls but not very helpful for an explosive tennis serve or use of a fork. This relates to the specificity of training, where performance gains are not transferable between dissimilar activities (see Chapter 7). In a fragmented form of rehabilitation, we would end up with a succession of new tasks, formed around these particular movement fragments, but ones which do not carry over any substantial benefits to the goal task.

Generally, training that employs movement fragmentation has not been shown to benefit the performance of the goal activity. For example, training that improves the local power at the ankle, or ankle and knee, fails to transfer to gains in vertical jumping, although this task depends on these neuromuscular components.[33] Exercises that isolate parts of the kicking action do not appear to transfer well to kicking

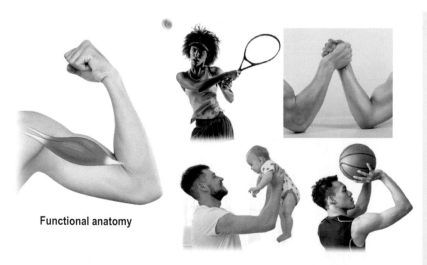

Functional anatomy

Same muscle, many recruitment patterns

FIGURE 8.4

Task-specific recruitment. The same muscle is used in all activities but recruitment patterns are unique to the task. Think control, not anatomy.

performance; training needs to involve the whole kicking action.[34] Training in isolated tasks, such as hip flexibility or trunk-strengthening activities, does not improve the economy of walking or running.[35] Core-specific exercises fail to improve the control of walking or sports performance.[36,37] In the elderly, resistance exercises have minimal influence on performance of daily activities, and in stroke patients functional improvements are more evident in whole-task practice.[38,39] (See Chapter 7 for more on training specificity).

There are two exceptions for using extra-functional localized exercise: in supporting repair and modulation of symptoms. In acute injuries, the affected joints/tissues can be singled out and exercised specifically to support the local repair process, e.g., sitting pendulum swings of the lower leg for an acute knee injury or post-surgery (see Chapter 14). However, this should be restricted to the initial inflammatory and proliferation phases. As the repair shifts toward the remodeling phase, movement should strive to resemble functional activities. As for modulation of symptoms, different forms of exercise can have an effect on symptoms, including area-specific exercises, such as limb-specific strengthening exercise for managing a symptomatic arthritic knee.[40] However, in terms of compliance and adherence, there may

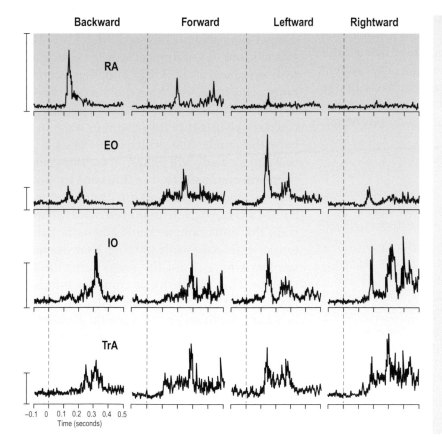

FIGURE 8.5

Recruitment specificity (electromyelogram) of anterior trunk muscles during bending. RA, rectus abdominis; EO, external oblique; IO, internal oblique; TrA, transversus abdominis. (After Carpenter MG, Tokuno CD, Thorstensson A, Cresswell AG. Differential control of abdominal muscles during multi-directional support-surface translations in man. Exper Brain Res. 2008;188:445.)

be greater benefit in management which is whole and functional (see Chapter 13).

In summary, practicing the task as a whole with a goal is faithful to the motor control processes underlying learning, recovery of movement control, and enhancement of skill performance. Using whole and goal movement means that the "injured expert" can train within their skill set. They can bypass practices that depend on dissociation and fragmentation of movement, practices which are likely to impede recovery rather than aid it. All forms of movement fragmentation are likely to be outside the person's experience and are therefore extra-functional in nature. Ultimately, these training approaches will fail to carry over meaningful benefits to the target activity (see specificity, Chapter 7). From a functional point of view, the most effective, efficient, and uncomplicated rehabilitation for the patient (and therapist) is to practice the affected tasks as a whole. The message at task-level rehabilitation is "*focus on the task and let the body organize the rest.*"

> **Beware of Frankensteinian rehabilitation:** in essence, the whole task cannot be recovered by "reverse engineering," using muscle-by-muscle, joint-by-joint rehabilitation, e.g., "strengthen this muscle, stretch the other". Such traditional training approaches can be likened to the creation of Frankenstein's monster: the attempt to reanimate a whole person by assembling a collection of different body parts. If Aristotle were present, he would surely remark that, "The task is greater than the sum of its muscles."

> A new training maxim: *"Integrate in order to coordinate"* (not *"fragment in order to integrate"*).
>
> In a functional approach, we rehabilitate the task and not "the muscle" – "practice the task and the body (muscle) will follow."

COMPONENT-FOCUSED REHABILITATION

So far, it has been proposed that, for recovering functionality, the focus should be on practicing the whole task. Now imagine a situation where a patient has walking difficulties following hip surgery. They are unable to sustain walking for more than a few minutes and, additionally, present with restricted stride length due to loss of hip flexibility. We can observe two distinct components of the task which have been affected: one is endurance, which is associated with duration of walking, and the second is range, associated with limitation in hip range of movement (ROM). In a task-level approach, we could simply instruct the patient to walk, in the hope that, under the principle of "practice the task and the body will follow," these two components will eventually recover. But what happens if only one does – if the walking distance recovers but the stride length remains restricted? To overcome this limitation, we could advise the patient to take wider steps while walking. Now, our intervention is focused on the range component of the task. This, in essence, is component-focused management, where the affected task components are identified and become the focus of the exercise intervention.[36] *Importantly, these components are always rehabilitated within the context of the affected task* (walking in this example). This is largely because all components are present in all tasks; however, each task has its unique component profile (Fig. 8.6A&B). For instance, the force profile of a tennis serve is very different to the force profile of lifting a cup of tea or lift-

ing a dumbbell. It means that these profiles are unique to the task and non-transferable between dissimilar activities (see specificity, Chapter 7).

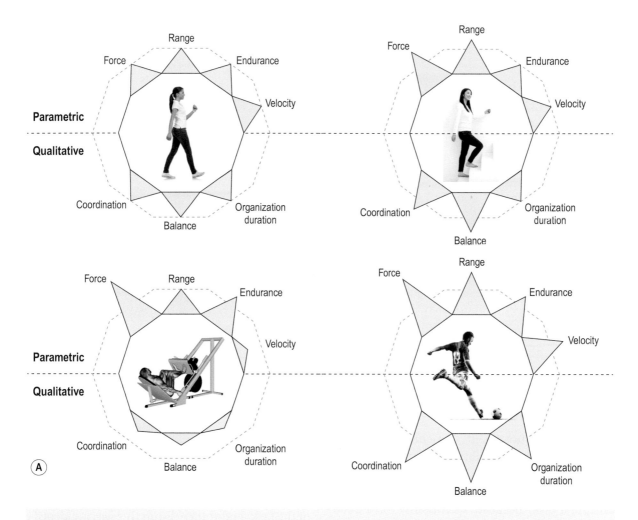

FIGURE 8.6

(A) An attempt to depict the task component profile in the legs during different activities in comparison to walking (dashed outline).

Continued

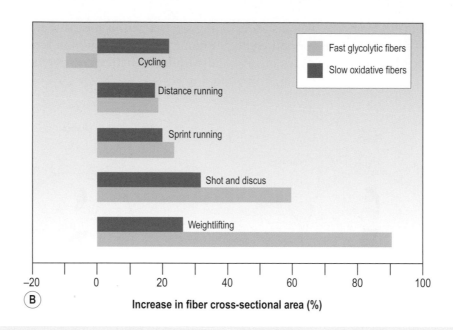

FIGURE 8.6 (CONTINUED)

(B) Different activities have their specific force-generation profiles. This can be observed to some extent in the ratio of the cross-sectional area between fast and slow muscle fibers in athletes participating in different sporting activities. Quadriceps biopsies were compared to sedentary controls. (After Goldspink G. Malleability of the motor system: a comparative approach. J Exper Biol. 1985;115:375–91.)

Task components

The task or movement components are the quantitative and qualitative features of skilled performance (Table 8.1).[41] It is about how much (*quantitative*) and how well (*qualitative*) we can execute a task. Because "quantitative" is a devil to pronounce we will use the term *parametric components* instead.

Parametric components can be explored by looking at a simple activity such as reaching and retrieving an object off a table. Several features of this activity can be modified without altering the nature of the task. It can be executed with varying degrees of force, such as in lifting a full or half-empty bottle, and performed at different speeds. The bottle can be placed close or further away on the table: range. This activity can be sustained for varying durations, depending on the nature of the task: endurance. From this we can identify four parametric components: *force, endurance, velocity,* and *movement range* (Table 8.1).[36]

The qualitative components can be explored using the same reaching example as above. In order to complete this task successfully, we need

Table 8.1 The task components and their role in performance

Parametric	Components	Description
	Force	Ability to generate and regulate force for successful performance of task
	Range	Ability to regulate range, perform full ranges in relation to successful performance of task
	Endurance	Ability to sustain task to completion (before experiencing fatigue – loss of force and velocity, and experiencing pain and exertion)
	Velocity	Ability to control speed / velocity of movement in relation to successful performance of task
Qualitative	Balance	Ability to accomplish task without falling over
	Coordination	Ability to synchronize different parts of body to produce movement that enables successful performance of task
	Organization duration	Ability to organize movement between two dissimilar activities without delay or disturbance to transition between them or goal task

to avoid falling over, so the balance component becomes important. If, at the same time, the hand was to manipulate an object, the fine harmonious working of the fingers/hand, as a whole, could be considered as fine coordination. The movement of the whole arm is single-limb coordination, and multi-limb coordination if we were synchronously using the other arm. Since the arms are attached to the rest of the body, the smooth integration of the limbs and the trunk can be viewed as whole-body coordination. Furthermore, we often tend to perform various tasks in succession. The reaching movement, if it took place while cooking, would be followed by actions such as holding, whisking, pouring, and so on. The ability to change seamlessly and rapidly between activities is termed organization duration – how long it takes to organize movement between two dissimilar tasks. From the above example, three qualitative components can be identified: *coordination*, *balance*, and *organization duration* (Table 8.1).[36]

A note on the force component: this component relates to the regulation of force required for successful performance of the task. Depending on the task, this can be through a spectrum ranging from maximum force generation, to the ability to fully relax the muscles, and every level in between. The ability to regulate and relax plays an important role in movement organization: for example, partial or full relaxation of paired muscle groups during movement, or reaching with a single arm when the other arm is resting unused (surround inhibition). The ability to regulate and switch off force is important in conditions where there is abnormal or excessive motor drive to muscles. This is seen in conditions such as muscle tension created by stress, and in dystonia and hypertonicity associated with central nervous system pathologies. An example of motor relaxation is discussed in Chapter 14, where a body scan relaxation, "micro relaxation," is used to manage chronic neck pain.

A note on balance: in musculoskeletal and pain conditions, single-leg (stance phase of walking) balance can be affected by discoordination of synergists on the affected side. This is different from central pathologies affecting the vestibular apparatus or cerebellum. In musculoskeletal injury, these centers/systems are still intact. Hence, the patient is usually able to perform single-leg activities on the non-affected side. A person with a central–vestibular balance deficit will be unsteady in a variety of weight-bearing activities, such as standing on both feet, single-leg balance on either side, or even getting up from sitting. Conveniently, there is no difference in the exercise approach for both forms of unsteadiness (see activity grading, Chapter 9).

Task components in peripheral and central pathology

The task components are affected to varying degrees in all conditions and can therefore become the focus of exercise prescription (Fig. 8.7).[36] The task components are regulated by motor control but also depend on a mixture of physical and physiological factors. Therefore, there is some relationship between how central and peripheral pathologies influence the two component groups. Understanding this relationship can help us tailor the exercise more precisely to the patient's condition.

Broadly, but not exclusively, musculoskeletal injuries or pain conditions are more likely to affect the parametric components. The task parameters are equally dependent on the physical integrity of the muscle and its motor control. For example, force generation is related to muscle hypertrophy, velocity and range to fascicle length, and endurance to mitochondrial activity. Yet, these components are also profoundly regulated by the motor system. Hence, the parametric components can be affected by muscle damage as well as CNS conditions (such as stroke), pain experiences, and movement fears.[42–45] For example, force and velocity of forward bending is decreased in acute or chronic low back pain but also in trunk movements that are perceived to be potentially harmful or painful.[46] The qualitative components can also be affected in musculoskeletal conditions. For example, injury is associated with discoordination of synergistic muscles groups local to the affected limb/area.[47,48]

Generally, the changes in the task components are more localized and less severe in musculoskeletal and pain conditions in comparison to CNS pathologies. This is largely because, in musculoskeletal conditions, the motor system is fully intact. The observed control changes are beneficial protective and restorative movement strategies: essentially, a foolproof tactic to restrain us from moving after an injury. The first line of protection is pain and fear of pain. Additionally, there is an attenuation of the four movement parameters to ensure that the individual gets the message to moderate their activities. So, loading of the damaged tissues is diminished by reducing force generation, speed, movement range, and the duration for which we

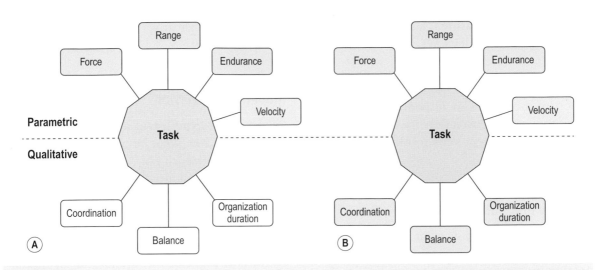

FIGURE 8.7

(A) Musculoskeletal injury, pain conditions, and movement fears tend to affect mostly the parametric components. (B) In central nervous system conditions, all components are likely to be affected, with more profound and diffuse changes, and a recovery which is often protracted and incomplete.

can sustain the activity (endurance). Later in the repair process, as the tissues begin to regain their tensile strength, these movement components are progressively challenged as the individual resumes their functional activities.

In CNS damage, both the qualitative and parametric components are dysregulated.[49–51] The qualitative components are largely dependent on motor processes but less so on peripheral contributions. They are, therefore, more likely to be influenced by CNS conditions. A person with stroke can have balance or coordination problems without a musculoskeletal injury. However, in CNS damage there is often profound dysregulation of the parametric components, such as muscle hyper- and hypotonicity. This has a knock-on effect on muscle physiology and morphology in the form of muscle atrophy, contractures, and so on.

Recovery of the task and its related components is more rapid and complete in musculoskeletal injuries (weeks), whereas it is slow, more diffuse throughout the body, and incomplete in CNS conditions.

MOVEMENT-FOCUSED REHABILITATION

Movement-focused rehabilitation is about "correctness of movement": identifying what is wrong and providing some form of movement re-education. In this approach, it is assumed that incorrect movement is detrimental to musculoskeletal health and physical performance. Movement re-education plays a major role in physical therapies, from advice on sitting and standing posture, bending and lifting instructions, lumbopelvic angles/rhythms, and scapular positioning, to sport performance styles, such as running or swimming techniques, and preventative measures, such as foot position in landing during ball games, and so on.

There are three key areas where movement is the focus of rehabilitation: protective organization of movement in response to injury and pain, movement correction for injury prevention, and movement repatterning to enhance task performance.

Movement organization in response to injury and pain

The most obvious movement reorganization is seen in the response to injury and pain – the antalgic postures and movements.[52,53] In these conditions, movement is reorganized in patterns that serve to reduce the physical stresses on the damaged or recovering tissues, largely in response to nociception and pain experience. So, is there any value in trying to modify the movement patterns associated with the injury response?

We have to assume that the body "knows best," that the antalgic behavior is the current "correct movement" in relation to the prevailing circumstances. For example, the gait pattern of a person with an acute knee injury or back pain represents the sum total of these internal and environmental variables. Hence, these patterns will be difficult to change without managing the underlying causes, such as resolution of repair or pain. This implies that, in acute conditions, the individual should be encouraged to remain active within their functional capacity, but to accept that the change in movement patterns is temporary, and likely to self-organize and normalize later on.

Movement-focused rehabilitation could be useful in situations where the antalgic gait or posture outlasts the symptomatic period; see

more below regarding movement reassurance versus re-education.

Permanent tissue damage and movement behavior

Symptomatic experiences are potent movement modulators, but what about damage without symptoms? At which point do asymptomatic tissue changes affect attainment of the task or the related movement patterns?

Movement control is highly influenced by pain and stiffness experiences, fear of movement, and conscious awareness of an injury.[46] However, in their absence, movement and functionality remain mostly unaffected, except in major tissue damage or neural conditions. Asymptomatic pathology without loss of functionality is ubiquitous throughout the body. This phenomenon has been observed in the feet (structural positional misalignments),[54,55] knees (as in arthritis, meniscal damage),[56,57] hips (such as labral tears, arthritis),[58-60] low back (disk and facet pathologies),[61,62] shoulders (capsular tears),[63,64] various tendinopathies,[65] and so on.

These "hidden" conditions rarely impact the individual's functional capacity unless they become symptomatic. A current example is my better half, who has a substantial asymptomatic medial meniscus tear. Every decade or so, and for no apparent reason, she has a knee pain episode, lasting 2–3 months, in which all weight-bearing activities are painful. Between these episodes she is able to carry out daily activities without any observable changes in her movement patterns, including regular jogging. This is despite the permanent tear. In such asymptomatic conditions, flareup periods are likely to recover by repair and, hence, may benefit from movement attenuation followed by gradual amplification as the symptoms subside. When asymptomatic, it might be better to leave it alone on the principle that "if it ain't symptomatic don't fix it."

But what about conditions that are expected to recover over a duration of a few weeks or months, such as movement limitations seen following knee immobilization or the stiff phase of frozen shoulder? Should we aim to prevent the elevation of the scapula in overhead reaching or correct the gait patterns following immobilization? Even in these slow-recovery conditions the principles discussed above apply. Manage the cause (loss of tissue extensibility) and let the body resolve the associated movement by practicing the affected task, as a whole, even if it seems "imperfect." It is assumed that, as tissues regain their extensibility, this will be reflected in more normalized movement patterns, keeping in mind that the pre-injury motor programs for walking remain intact. These motor programs are robust and can remain unchanged for many years, even without practice. Hence, they are likely to survive a few weeks or months of altered activity. The movement intervention for walking could be to "take wider steps until you feel a bit of a stretch behind the knee," and so on. For the frozen shoulder, the instruction could be to favor the affected arm and to challenge end-ranges during daily activities, such as reaching and retrieving from higher shelves. The instruction to the patient could be "reach until you feel a stretch or discomfort." In these walking and reaching examples, the focus of rehabilitation is the range component. This functional stretching approach is described in more detail in Lederman (2013).[66]

There are also the movement adaptations associated with extensive, irreparable, and permanent musculoskeletal or neurological damage, such as complete tendon tears or foot drop. These altered movement patterns are the outcome, the adaptation to an unrecoverable condition. Without improving the underlying cause, the chances of normalizing the movement are very slim.

The take-away points so far are: regardless of the condition's time scale or severity, alteration in movement patterns is an outcome and not the cause, an adaptation and the best solution under the current circumstances. The message to the patient is clear: practice the whole task – do not worry too much about how you are performing it. As the therapist, consider this: if movement re-education is introduced, there is only 20–60% chance that the patient will remember the instructions, a 50% chance that they will perform it correctly, and a 50% chance that they will ever practice it – a bit of a non-starter.

Movement reassurance versus movement re-education

It is not uncommon for patients to retain their protective movement strategies long after they have recovered from their condition. They can be maintained by psychological factors rather than true structural or neurological damage.[46] Psychological factors include fear of pain, anxieties about re-injury, and catastrophizing about future disability.[67] Additional factors are excessive internal focusing and hypervigilance on the workings of the body and being overprotective about minor, commonly experienced discomfort.[68,69]

This phenomenon of using "redundant" protective movement strategies can be observed in individuals who have experienced back pain in the past but are presently symptom-free. Through previous pain experiences and a sprinkling of misinformation, they will employ an antalgic protective posture in a variety of daily activities. They often perform tasks such as reaching, bending, and sitting with a stiff, straight back in the erroneous belief that they are protecting their back.[70] This misconception sustains them in the mindset that they are permanent back pain sufferers, even at times when they are pain-free. After three or four decades of research into back pain causes and management, we can confidently say that there is no association between posture, biomechanics, movement, and back pain.[71] Hence, they can safely move, stand, sit, and operate in any way they wish.[72,73] With this in mind, these fears can be challenged in clinic. An approach I often use is to stand in front of the patient, slightly further away than their arm's reach. I put my hands forward and instruct them to reach and tap them several times with both hands. I then move my hands to a different position, which they have to follow and tap (Fig. 13.1A–F). As they gain confidence, I position my hand further away, encouraging them to bend and twist to reach, challenging them to use the misconceived "wrong/bad/dangerous" spinal movements. I often use this form of movement reassurance in clinic – a "de-education" rather than movement re-education (see Chapter 13).

> **Message to the anxious patient:** "enjoy your body, don't be afraid of it."

Performance modification and injury prevention/minimization

Enhancing performance and providing exercise for minimizing injury is somewhat outside the remit of this book; however, these topics are included to address questions about movement re-education and exercise prescription.

Both enhancement of skill and movement repatterning for injury prevention are largely motor learning phenomena. For most of our patients, their skills have been acquired over many years. Changing these tenacious motor programs – e.g., a new batting or swimming stroke – is likely to take several weeks to months. This raises the issue of timing. When is it suitable to introduce movement repatterning after an injury? An important consideration is the patient's capacity to learn during the period of recovery. Re-forming familiar skillful activities requires a substantial and prolonged investment in practice, an intervention which may not be suitable for a person recovering from a musculoskeletal injury. They are in pain or discomfort, with reduced physical capacity, and are anxious and psychologically focused on the effects of the injury on their life. Perhaps management that aims to enhance performance or minimize injury could be postponed until the individual is fully recovered and functional, a time more suitable to take on new learning challenges.

SUMMARY

- This chapter has explored task-, component-, and movement-focused rehabilitation.

- In task-focused rehabilitation the affected activity is practiced as a whole.

- In component rehabilitation the focus is on particular elements of the task, such as balance, force, endurance, and so on.

- Movement-level rehabilitation focuses on correcting or modifying the task-related movement patterns.

Task-focused practice – whole and goal

- The whole body is organized specifically to support the task. The task should be practiced as whole and goal.

- Management that focuses internally on body parts, muscles, or joints favors decoupling the movement from the task and further fragmenting it. This tends to degrade performance or may even change the treatment goals.

Task components

- There are two groups of task components: parametric and qualitative.

- The parametric components are: force, endurance, velocity, and movement range.

- The qualitative components are: coordination, balance, and organization duration.

- Musculoskeletal and pain conditions and movement-related fears tend to affect mainly the parametric group.

- The qualitative components are largely affected in CNS conditions.

- The task parameters can be attenuated or amplified in line with the individual's condition.

Movement re-education

- The ability to perform the task is more important than the quality of its movement.

- The current movement strategy is the body's best solution under the current circumstances.

- A change in movement pattern is an outcome, but rarely the cause of the condition.

Chapter 8

- Antalgic movements or postures represent the best solution under the circumstances – there is no need to modify them.

- Movement is organized in response to symptomatic experiences but not necessarily by asymptomatic pathology.

- Symptom management may be more important than movement repatterning.

- Changing the task-related movement can be challenging, particularly if the activity has become habitual.

- Individuals who have movement-related anxieties may benefit more from movement reassurance than movement re-education.

References

1. Magill RA. Motor learning concepts and applications. Iowa: William C Brown; 1985.

2. Elliott D, Helsen WF, Chua R. A century later: Woodworth's (1899) two-component model of goal-directed aiming. Psychol Bull. 2001;127:342.

3. Prinz W. Perception and action planning. Eur J Cogn Psychol. 1997;9:129–54.

4. Elsner B, Hommel B. Effect anticipation and action control. J Exp Psychol Hum Percept Perform. 2001;27:229.

5. Pereira J, Ofner P, Schwarz A, Sburlea AI, Müller-Putz GR. EEG neural correlates of goal-directed movement intention. Neuroimage. 2017;149:129–40.

6. Hommel B, Müsseler J, Aschersleben G, Prinz W. The theory of event coding (TEC): a framework for perception and action planning. Behav Brain Sci. 2001;24:849.

7. McNevin NH, Wulf G, Carlson C. Effects of attentional focus, self-control, and dyad training on motor learning: implications for physical rehabilitation. Phys Ther. 2000;80:373–85.

8. Beilock SL, Carr TH, MacMahon C, Starkes JL. When paying attention becomes counterproductive: impact of divided versus skill-focused attention on novice and experienced performance of sensorimotor skills. J Exp Psychol Appl. 2002;8:6–16.

9. Wulf G, McConnel N, Gärter M, Schwarz A. Enhancing the learning of sport skills through external-focus feedback. J Mot Behav. 2002;34:171–82.

10. Zachry T, Wulf G, Mercer J, Bezodis N. Increased movement accuracy and reduced EMG activity as the result of adopting an external focus of attention. Brain Res Bull. 2005;67:304–9.

11. Marchant D, Greig M, Scott C. Attentional focusing instructions influence force production and muscular activity during isokinetic elbow flexions. J Strength Cond Res. 2009;23:2358–66.

12. Vance J, Wulf G, Töllner T, McNevin N, Mercer J. EMG activity as a function of the performer's focus of attention. J Mot Behav. 2004;36:450–9.

13. Wulf G, Lauterbach B, Toole T. The learning advantages of an external focus of attention in golf. Res Q Exerc Sport. 1999;70:120–6.

14. Wulf G, McConnel N, Gärtner M, Schwarz A. Enhancing the learning of sport skills through external-focus feedback. J Motor Behav. 2002;34:171–82.

15. Wulf G, Wächter S, Wortmann S. Attentional focus in motor skill learning: do females benefit from an external focus?. Women Sport Phys Act J. 2003;12:37–52.

16. McNevin NH, Shea CH, Wulf G. Increasing the distance of an external focus of attention enhances learning. Psychol Res. 2003;67:22–9.

17. Brown SH, Vera-Garcia FJ, McGill SM. Effects of abdominal muscle coactivation on the externally preloaded trunk: variations in motor control and its effect on spine stability. Spine. 2006;31:E387–93.

18. Lederman E. The myth of core stability. J Bodyw Move Ther. 2010;14:84–98.

19. Gray R. Differences in attentional focus associated with recovery from sports injury: does injury induce an internal focus? J Sport Exerc Psychol. 2015;37:607–16.

20. Laufer Y, Rotem-Lehrer N, Ronen Z, Khayutin G, Rozenberg I. Effect of attention focus on acquisition and retention of postural control following ankle sprain. Arch Phys Med Rehab. 2007;88:105–8.

21. Landers MR, Wulf G, Wallmann HW, Guadagnoli M. An external focus of attention attenuates balance impairment in Parkinson's disease. Physiotherapy. 2005;91:152–85.

22. Wulf G, Landers M, Lewthwaite R, Töllner T. External focus instructions reduce postural instability in individuals with Parkinson disease. Phys Ther. 2009;89:162–8.

23. Fasoli SE, Trombly CA, Tickle-Degnan L, Verfaelie MH. Effect of instructions on functional reach in persons with and without cerebrovascular accident. Am J Occup Ther. 2002;56:380–90.

24. Patla AE, Ishac MG, Winter DA. Anticipatory control of center of mass and joint stability during voluntary arm movement from a standing posture: interplay between active and passive control. Exper Brain Res. 2002;143:318–27.

25. Beck S, Hallett M. Surround inhibition in the motor system. Exp Brain Res. 2011;210:165–72.

26. Doemges F, Rack PM. Task-dependent changes in the response of human wrist joints to mechanical disturbance. J Physiol. 1992;447:575–85.

27. McGill SM, Kippers V. Transfer of loads between lumbar tissues during the flexion-relaxation phenomenon. Spine. 1994;19:2190–6.

28. Decker MJ, Tokish JM, Ellis HB, Torry MR, Hawkins RJ. Subscapularis muscle activity during selected rehabilitation exercises. Am J Sports Med. 2003;31:126–34.

29. Hore J, McCloskey DI, Taylor JL. Task-dependent changes in gain of the reflex response to imperceptible perturbations of joint position in man. J Physiol. 1990;429:309–21.

30. Carpenter MG, Tokuno CD, Thorstensson A, Cresswell AG. Differential control of abdominal muscles during multi-directional support-surface translations in man. Exper Brain Res. 2008;188:445.

31. Andersson EA, Oddsson LI, Grundström H, Nilsson J, Thorstensson A. EMG activities of the quadratus lumborum and erector spinae muscles during flexion-relaxation and other motor tasks. Clin Biomech (Bristol, Avon). 1996;11:392–400.

32. Kavcic N, Grenier S, McGill SM. Determining the stabilizing role of individual torso muscles during rehabilitation exercises. Spine. 2004;29:1254–65.

33. Leirdal S, Roeleveld K, Ettema G. Coordination specificity in strength and power training. Int J Sports Med. 2008;29:225–31.

34. Young WB, Rath DA. Enhancing foot velocity in football kicking: the role of strength training. J Strength Cond Res. 2011;25:561–6.

35. Godges JJ, MacRae PG, Engelke KA. Effects of exercise on hip range of motion, trunk muscle performance, and gait economy. Phys Ther.1993;73:468–77.

36. Lederman E. Neuromuscular rehabilitation in manual and physical therapy. Edinburgh: Churchill Livingstone; 2010.

37. Wirth K, Hartmann H, Mickel C, Szilvas E, Keiner M, Sander A. Core stability in athletes: a critical analysis of current guidelines. Sports Med. 2017;47:401–14.

38. Liu C-J, Shiroy DM, Jones LY, Clark DO. Systematic review of functional training on muscle strength, physical functioning, and activities of daily living in older adults. Eur Rev Aging Phys Activ. 2014;11:144.

39. Veerbeek JM, van Wegen E, van Peppen R, van der Wees PJ, Hendriks E, Rietberg M. What is the evidence for physical therapy poststroke? A systematic review and meta-analysis. PLoS One 2014;9:e87987.

40. Fransen M, McConnell S, Harmer AR, Van der Esch M, Simic M, Bennell KL. Exercise for osteoarthritis of the knee. Cochrane Database Syst Rev. 2015 Jan 8;1:CD004376.

41. Fleishman EA. Toward a taxonomy of human performance. Am Psychol. 1975;30:1127.

42. Van Lent ME, Drost MR, van den Wildenberg FA. EMG profiles of ACL-deficient patients during walking: the influence of mild fatigue. Int J Sports Med. 1994;15:508–14.

43. Shirado O, Ito T, Kaneda K, Strax TE. Concentric and eccentric strength of trunk muscles: influence of test postures on strength and characteristics of patients with chronic low-back pain. Arch Phys Med Rehabil. 1995;76:604–11.

44. Kamper DG, Fischer HC, Cruz EG, Rymer WZ. Weakness is the primary contributor to finger impairment in chronic stroke. Arch Phys Med Rehab. 2006;87:1262–9.

45. Stokes M, Young A. The contribution of reflex inhibition to arthrogenous muscle weakness. Clin Sci. 1984;67:7–14.

46. Thomas JS, France CR, Lavender SA, Johnson MR. Effects of fear of movement on spine velocity and acceleration after recovery from low back pain. Spine. 2008;33:564–70.

47. St-Onge N, Duval N, Yahia L, Feldman AG. Interjoint coordination in lower limbs in patients with a rupture of the anterior cruciate ligament of the knee joint. Knee Surg Sports Traumatol Arthrosc. 2004;12:203–16.

48. Cholewicki J, Panjabi MM, Khachatryan A. Stabilizing function of trunk flexor-extensor muscles around a neutral spine posture. Spine. 1997;22:2207-12.

49. Mihaltchev P, Archambault PS, Feldman AG, Levin MF. Control of double-joint arm posture in adults with unilateral brain damage. Exper Brain Res. 2005;163:468–86.

50. Beer RF, Dewald JP, Rymer WZ. Deficits in the coordination of multijoint arm movements in patients with hemiparesis: evidence for disturbed control of limb dynamics. Exp Brain Res. 2000;131:305–19.

51. Tedroff K, Knutson LM, Soderberg GL. Synergistic muscle activation during maximum voluntary contractions in children with and without spastic

cerebral palsy. Dev Med Child Neurol. 2006;48:789–96.

52. Ozveren MF, Bilge T, Barut S, Eras M. Combined approach for far-lateral lumbar disc herniation. Neurol Med Chir. 2004;44:118–23.

53. Crosbie J, Green T, Refshauge K. Effects of reduced ankle dorsi-flexion following lateral ligament sprain on temporal and spatial gait parameters. Gait Posture. 1999;9:167–72.

54. Garbalosa JC, McClure MH, Catlin PA, Wooden M. The frontal plane relationship of the forefoot to the rearfoot in an asympto-matic population. J Orthop Sports Phys Ther. 1994;20:200–6.

55. Jarvis HL, Nester CJ, Bowden PD, Jones RK. Challenging the foundations of the clinical model of foot function: further evidence that the root model assessments fail to appropriately classify foot function. J Foot Ankle Res. 2017;10:7.

56. Clauw DJ. Diagnosing and treating chronic musculoskeletal pain based on the underlying mechanism(s). Best Pract Res Clin Rheumatol. 2015;29:6–19.

57. Bedson J, Croft PR. The dis-cordance between clinical and radiographic knee osteoarthritis: a systematic search and summary of the literature. BMC Musculo-skelet Disord. 2008;9:116–27.

58. Schmitz MR, Campbell SE, Fajardo RS, Kadrmas WR. Identification of acetabular labral pathological changes in asymptomatic volunteers using optimized, noncontrast 1.5-T magnetic resonance imaging. Am J Sports Med. 2012;40:1337–41.

59. Lee AJ, Armour P, Thind D, Coates MH, Kang AC.

The prevalence of acetabular labral tears and associated pathology in a young asympto-matic population. Bone Joint J. 2015;97:623–7.

60. Heerey JJ, Kemp JL, Mosler AB, Jones DM, Pizzari T, Souza RB, et al. What is the prevalence of imaging-defined intra-articular hip pathologies in people with and without pain? A systematic review and meta-analysis. Br J Sports Med. 2018;52:581–93.

61. Boos N, Rieder R, Schade V, Spratt KF, Semmer N, Aebi M. Volvo Award in clinical sci-ences. The diagnostic accuracy of magnetic resonance imaging, work perception, and psycho-social factors in identifying symptomatic disc herniations. Spine. 1995;20:2613–25.

62. Brinjikji W, Luetmer PH, Com-stock B, Bresnahan BW, Chen LE, Deyo RA, et al. Systematic literature review of imaging features of spinal degeneration in asymptomatic populations. Am J Neuroradiol. 2015;36:811–16.

63. Sher JS, Uribe JW, Posada A, Murphy BJ, Zlatkin MB. Abnormal findings on magnetic resonance images of asympto-matic shoulders. J Bone Joint Surg Am. 1995;77:10–15.

64. Girish G. Ultrasound of the shoulder: asymptomatic findings in men. Am J Roent-genol. 2011;197:W713–19.

65. van Sterkenburg MN, van Dijk CN. Mid-portion Achil-les tendinopathy: why painful? An evidence-based philosophy. Knee Surg Sports Traumatol Arthrosc. 2011;19:1367–75.

66. Lederman E. Therapeutic stretching: towards a functional

approach. Edinburgh: Elsevier Health Sciences; 2013.

67. Parr JJ, Borsa PA, Fillingim RB, Tillman MD, Manini TM, Gregory CM, et al. Pain-related fear and catastrophizing predict pain intensity and disability independently using an induced muscle injury model. J Pain. 2012;13:370–8.

68. Crombez G, Van Damme S, Eccleston C. Hypervigilance to pain: an experimental and clin-ical analysis. Pain. 2005;116:4–7.

69. Herbert MS, Goodin BR, Pero ST 4th, Schmidt JK, Sotolongo A, Bulls HW, et al. Pain hyper-vigilance is associated with greater clinical pain severity and enhanced experimen-tal pain sensitivity among adults with symptomatic knee osteoarthritis.Ann Behav Med. 2014;48:50-60.

70. Verbeek JH, Martimo KP, Kuijer PP, Karppinen J, Viikari-Juntura E, Takala EP. Proper manual handling tech-niques to prevent low back pain, a Cochrane systematic review. Work. 2012;41:2299–301.

71. Lederman E. The fall of the pos-tural-structural-biomechanical model in manual and physical therapies: exemplified by lower back pain. J Bodyw Move Ther. 2011;15:131–8.

72. Nolan D. What do physiothera-pists and manual handling advisors consider the safest lifting posture, and do back beliefs influence their choice? Musculoskelet Sci Pract. 2018;33:35-40.

73. O'Sullivan K. What do physi-otherapists consider to be the best sitting spinal posture? Man Ther. 2012;17:432–7.

Chapter 9

Contents
Activity grading within a functional approach

Activity grading is all about easing ourselves back to activity. It involves a stepwise increase or decrease in intensity, demands, or complexity placed on an activity.

We all are natural experts in activity grading. This course of action is embedded within our training practices and recovery behavior; it is what most people do during learning, when they are practicing to enhance their performance, or when they are injured. If you sprain your ankle, initially there will be a period of activity attenuation associated with the repair protection phase. This will be followed by the functional restorative phase, during which there is gradual resumption in walking duration, distance, speed, and stride length. Essentially, these behavioral activity grading patterns inform exercise prescription.

So, how do we construct a safe graded management plan? Where does it start and when does it end? Well, it's all about patients' goals, experimentation, and some creativity.

CONSTRUCTING AN ACTIVITY GRADING SCHEDULE

The activity grading plan commences by inviting the individual to identify their functional recovery goals. These can be a mixture of activities from the shared and unique repertoire (Fig. 9.1): for example, walking and returning to play tennis. Generally, the management commences with the less physically demanding, shared repertoire (walking) and progresses to the unique repertoire, which contains the individual's sporting activities (tennis). This is followed by setting the start and end-point for rehabilitation. These markers are usually defined by the patient's pre- and post-injury capacity in the selected activity. For example, if they were able to walk for 1 hour pre-injury and currently only able to walk for 5 minutes, these durations are set as the start and end-point of rehabilitation. The grading is then loosely constructed around an 8–9-week period, which is roughly the time

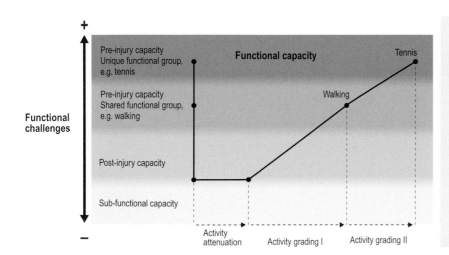

FIGURE 9.1

Activity grading is set within the pre- and post-injury capacity. Generally, it starts with the less challenging daily activities within the shared repertoire and then progresses to the more demanding unique repertoire that often contains sports activities.

in which the shared activities are expected to recover (Fig. 9.2). However, the length of the rehabilitation period can change, depending on many variables, such as extent of injury, tissue affected, surgical procedure, patient's goals, and so on.

Each week on the plan represents a stepwise increase in exposure to the activity (Fig. 9.3). Variables such as distance or time and daily frequency can be set in advance and modified when necessary. Depending on the nature of the condition, the increase can be by any proportion: increments of perhaps 5 minutes or similar. If it all goes well, after 3-4 weeks, for example, the increase can escalate to 10-minute increments, and so on. If, at any point, the activity results in worsening of the condition or is unsustainable, it can be scaled back to a less challenging activity level. This stage can be consolidated over the next 1–3 weeks, then re-evaluated and grading resumed if considered safe (Fig. 9.4). The grading plan can be applied as a stand-alone for any activity within the functional range. For example, a patient may wish to resume jogging after leg injury or surgery with a stated goal of recovering their 1-hour running capacity. The grading can start with their current ability of, e.g., 5 minutes, repeated two or three times a week and, if safe, increased weekly by 5–10-minute increments, and so on.

Name		Start date							
	Week 1 (post-protective/attenuation phase)	**Week 2**	**Week 3**	**Week 4**	**Week 5**	**Week 6**	**Week 7**	**Week 8**	Add or remove weeks as necessary
Identify patient's primary recovery goal (e.g., walking)	Establish baseline capacity for chosen activity							Establish goal capacity (usually the patient's pre-injury capacity)	
Patient's secondary recovery goal (e.g., tennis)	Establish baseline capacity							Establish goal capacity	
Add recovery goals, if needed	Etc.							Etc.	

FIGURE 9.2

An example of activity grading.

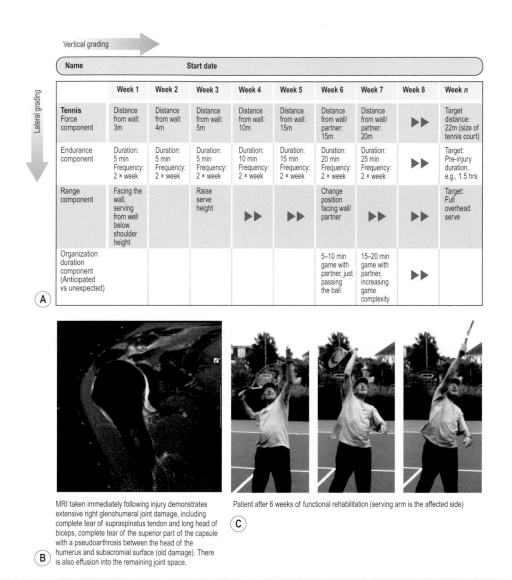

Vertical grading →

Lateral grading ↓

Name						Start date			
	Week 1	Week 2	Week 3	Week 4	Week 5	Week 6	Week 7	Week 8	Week n
Tennis Force component	Distance from wall: 3m	Distance from wall: 4m	Distance from wall: 5m	Distance from wall: 10m	Distance from wall: 15m	Distance from wall/partner: 15m	Distance from wall/partner: 20m	▶▶	Target distance: 22m (size of tennis court)
Endurance component	Duration: 5 min Frequency: 2 × week	Duration: 5 min Frequency: 2 × week	Duration: 5 min Frequency: 2 × week	Duration: 10 min Frequency: 2 × week	Duration: 15 min Frequency: 2 × week	Duration: 20 min Frequency: 2 × week	Duration: 25 min Frequency: 2 × week	▶▶	Target: Pre-injury duration, e.g., 1.5 hrs
Range component	Facing the wall, serving from well below shoulder height		Raise serve height	▶▶	▶▶	Change position facing wall/partner	▶▶	▶▶	Target: Full overhead serve
Organization duration component (Anticipated vs unexpected)						5–10 min game with partner, just passing the ball	15–20 min game with partner, increasing game complexity	▶▶	

(A)

MRI taken immediately following injury demonstrates extensive right glenohumeral joint damage, including complete tear of supraspinatus tendon and long head of biceps, complete tear of the superior part of the capsule with a pseudoarthrosis between the head of the humerus and subacromial surface (old damage). There is also effusion into the remaining joint space.

(B)

Patient after 6 weeks of functional rehabilitation (serving arm is the affected side)

(C)

FIGURE 9.3

Activity grading for a tennis player after shoulder injury. (A) The patient is past the protective phase and at the start of the restorative phase. The overall duration and grading change, depending on several factors. (B) Due to the extent of damage, the patient's age (75), and other health issues, it was decided to rehabilitate the shoulder using a non-surgical route: in this case, a functional approach. In the first 2 weeks the patient was in severe pain, with extensive hematoma in the arm and loss of arm functionality. This early protective phase of repair was managed with pendulum exercises (see Fig. 14.4A–B). At the end of 2 weeks the patient was mostly pain-free but had complete loss of arm functionality. The shared functionality was challenged using daily activities (see text and Figs 14.9A–H, 14.5A–C, 14.6A–F, 14.7A–B, and 14.8A–H). Tennis was used as the remedial exercise for that activity (A). (C) 6 weeks post-injury, the patient was fully functional and played his first game of tennis. The patient and his coach estimated that he was playing at 85% of his pre-injury capacity. Remarkably, he is still playing tennis 10 years later.

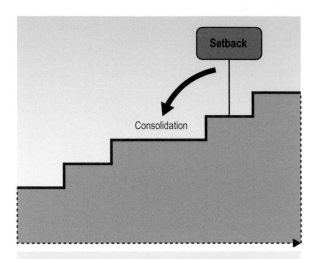

FIGURE 9.4
Vertical grading of activities is associated with amplification of the task components. Each step represents a week. If, at one point, there is a setback, the management can be scaled back to an earlier level which is considered safe.

GRADING FORMS

Grading of any activity can take several forms (Table 9.1). A vertical grading is used to challenge the task components, usually by a gradual increase in the intensity of the activity, such as the duration/distance of walking, running, rowing, playing tennis, and so on. Often, vertical grading is introduced at the beginning of rehabilitation and used for challenging the four task parameters.

A lateral task grading introduces several related activities from the individual's functional repertoire in a sequence. This can be within the shared group – for example, walking progressing to climbing stairs; or from the shared to the unique repertoire – walking to climbing stairs and then progressing to running. Often, lateral grading is introduced when the base activity (say, walking) has improved sufficiently to support the succeeding activity.

Table 9.1 Grading patterns		
Grading	**Pattern**	**Example: Soccer player with a leg injury**
Vertical	Challenging task components within a single activity	Walk at comfortable speed and then walk faster Increase stride length
Lateral	Adding activities that share regional functionality (see Chapter 2)	Walk, stairs and then play soccer
Subskill integration	Single subskill to mixing several subskills	Walking and dribbling a ball, passing ball between feet, running and kicking a ball
Organization duration	Anticipated to unexpected challenges	Kick ball to a wall then passing to a partner

	Week 1	Week 2	Week 3	Week 4	Week 5	Week 6	Week 7	Week 8	Week 9	Week 10	Week 11	Week 12
Tennis	Start here											
Running				Start here								
Cycling								Start here				

FIGURE 9.5
Lateral grading and staggering goal activities.

Subskill integration is another form of lateral activity grading. Many sports activities contain a number of subskills, in particular team sports such as basketball where the player has to switch from running and dribbling, and passing the ball to taking shots and defending. Here, the grading progresses vertically in the least demanding subskill (running and dribbling) and then laterally to the more physically demanding skill set (such as hook shot).

Lateral grading often contains a staggered pattern where activities are introduced sequentially with a "safety" gap between them (Fig. 9.5). For example, a patient expresses a wish to improve walking, running, and cycling. All these activities can be staggered, starting off with the least demanding and most essential activity, such as walking. Then, 3 weeks later, running is added and, some time later, cycling is reintroduced. The sequence is decided by the patient, according to their priorities. The time gap between the activities is mostly decided with safety in mind and in relation to improvements in the preceding activity.

Grading can be viewed as an experiment; there is no rule of thumb. The planning requires flexibility and should provide the patient with choice in activity prioritizing and planning the management particulars. However, if it is unreasonable, be ready to step in and negotiate the plan to a safe and realistic level.

GRADING THE PARAMETRIC COMPONENTS

The task components can also be graded up or down, depending on the presenting condition. As discussed elsewhere, the main consideration is that they are challenged within the affected activities. Generally, the grading starts off with the components most affected. Activities that are performed by the person by themselves (e.g., walking) can be practiced by the person on their own. Team activities can be self-practiced and later progress to training with a coach or another player.

The first component grading example is from the shared activities: grading walking for a patient who is in the restorative recovery phase following a lower limb injury or surgery. From this information we can already start to construct the exercise management: firstly, the rehabilitation will be in the direction of grading amplification; secondly, this being a musculoskeletal condition, it is expected that the parametric components will be mostly impacted; and thirdly, the law of specificity decrees that the exercise has to be managed within the goal task – that is, walking. So, we are looking at vertical grading of force, endurance, movement range, and velocity within walking. Force can be amplified by increasing the speed of walking, stepping over obstacles, and hill walking; endurance by increasing the time spent walking; and range of motion by increasing the stride length.

Once there is progress in walking, the question is "what next?" At this point, lateral activity grading can be introduced – but which activities? As discussed in Chapter 2, the lower limb is used in the context of what the individual does with their legs within their environment: all weight-bearing activities such as getting into and out of chairs and using stairs. These activities can be added and vertically graded. Sit-to-stand force can be graded by progressively lowering the height of the seat (starting with a cushion or two to raise the height and then removing them and, preferably, rising from sitting without use of the arms). Further escalation of force can be introduced by leaning sideways towards the affected side while getting up from sitting, and so on (see Chapter 14). Vertical force and endurance grading for stair climbing can include the number of stairs climbed, the rate of climbing, use of the arms to winch oneself up, and then free stair walking, and so on.

Now, let's imagine that the person described above with the leg condition has been rehabilitated for walking and is keen to recover playing tennis. Is it possible to construct a graded leg recovery program from an activity which is associated with upper limb movements, such as tennis? Yes, it is. Tennis is a whole-body

recruitment phenomenon; hence, it can be employed to rehabilitate the lower limbs but equally is useful to manage a person with a back or upper limb condition. A person recovering from a back injury, who happens to be a tennis player, can use tennis as the remedial exercise. No need for back-specific exercises (they do not really exist as a unique movement group – almost all human activities involve the trunk/spine). So, what does a remedial tennis grading program look like?

Let's for a minute imagine that 2–3 weeks have passed since the onset of the condition. It is expected that the patient is within the early part of the restorative stage. Here, too, the management introduces vertical grading of the parametric components within playing tennis. With this in mind, grading can start by serving the ball against a wall, e.g., 2–3 meters away (or facing another player or the trainer). The force component can be amplified by serving from greater distances – 4, 5, or 6 meters in each subsequent week, and so on. This grading challenge would also cover the velocity component of the serve. The endurance component can be graded by keeping the distance but increasing the activity's duration, again, starting at 5, then 10 and 15 minutes in successive weeks, and so on. The range component of the serve can be manipulated by changing the standing position: facing the wall, standing with either side at 90° to the wall, or serving to different locations on the wall (see Fig. 9.3A).

GRADING THE QUALITATIVE COMPONENTS

A quick reminder: we are now looking at grading components such as coordination, balance, and organization time. The starting point is the basic grading principles described above: the direction of grading – amplification or attenuation; the relationship of the components affected to the condition; and keeping the grading within the task.

Generally, the qualitative components are profoundly affected in central nervous system (CNS) conditions and neglect or detraining, as in immobilization. Comparatively, in musculoskeletal injuries they are mildly and temporarily affected, with some broad exceptions such as extensive musculoskeletal damage and peripheral nerve injury. Hence, grading of the qualitative is usually in the direction of amplification. Additionally, amplification in this component group means some form of increase in complexity of the challenge, rather than in its intensity.

Grading balance challenge

Balance is surprising. The more we focus on our body, the worse our balance performance is. It seems that the further away the focus is from the body and out of consciousness, the better the balance performance is (see Chapter 8). This phenomenon is present both in healthy individuals and in those suffering from CNS damage. Single-leg balance tends to degrade when focusing internally on the position and activity of the foot in comparison to focusing on some distant point away from the body. Stroke patients display better balance performance when they are given an additional task while walking, such as passing a ball from one hand to the other. That makes some sense. Balance is always there in the background of our awareness, no matter how complex the task is. We rarely notice it unless we trip. So, how do we grade and rehabilitate balance, particularly, without drawing attention to it?

Often in rehabilitation, balance ability is challenged by a static single-leg stance; but here is a pitfall. Generally, single-leg balance has a transitional role within the functional repertoire, such as the stance phase of walking or single-leg stance when kicking a soccer ball. Otherwise, humans rarely stand on a single leg, unless they set out to challenge it with activities such as yoga or tai chi, or are tested for sobriety. More important is the dynamic, transient single-leg stance seen in activities such as walking and climbing stairs. This ability can be graded by encouraging the person to spend more time on the affected side. It can be graded by lowering the pace of walking, increasing the stride length, stepping with the unaffected leg over a low and then a raised obstacle, and walking and turning while in the stance phase, on the affected side (see Chapter 14). For safety, this activity should be practiced initially with some form of support, such as walking along a wall in a hallway or around a dinner table, and so on. Eventually, balance can be challenged by going up and down stairs slowly – aided (!) and then unaided.

If the person happens to be a soccer player, the balance challenge could follow the exercise described previously: standing on the affected side while dribbling the ball between the inner and outer step of the unaffected foot (attempting to keep the unaffected foot from contacting the ground). Dynamic single-leg balance can be drastically challenged by placing the ball at various distances from the player and kicking it with the unaffected side.

A note on balance specificity: there is no transfer in balance ability between different activities, including walking and standing. Balance has to be practiced and graded individually within each task.

Finally, how do we draw the person's attention away from the balance activity? Keep them focused externally – "eyes on the goal" – by practicing the balance challenges within task.

Grading coordination

Firstly, let's examine what we mean by coordination: something like the ability to complete a task successfully by synchronizing different parts of the body in a movement which is efficient and within a path of least deviation. Discoordination is the opposite – the inability to complete the task successfully due to some failure in synchronization. Now, how can we grade that? The answer is that probably we can't. The coordination for typing does not transfer to playing the piano (see Chapter 7). Equally, when a person trains for lumbopelvic control on the floor, it does not transfer to coordination in standing or walking. In stroke patients, single-limb coordination practice does not transfer to multi-limb coordination. Multi-limb coordination has to be practiced as a whole and unfragmented (see Chapter 7). Basically, coordination is another component that is highly specific and has to be practiced as a whole within the affected activities.

A note on expected and unexpected challenges and organization duration component

Every aspect of our activities can be graded, even organization duration. As a reminder, this component represents the duration it takes to change between dissimilar activities, such as sit-to-stand or walk and turn, and so on. There are two principal grading methods for organization duration: practicing by ourselves or with others.

Organization duration can be challenged by practicing two or more activities in succession, such as walking and then turning, or running with a ball and then sidestepping. The grading here is in the minimization of the transition duration spent between the two activities.

Generally, activities which we carry out on our own are not as taxing in terms of movement organization as activities that are performed with others. So, the next grading level is to introduce unexpected challenges by training with a companion. On our own, we have ample time to prepare for the expected, such as transitioning between walking and climbing stairs, or practicing basketball shots by ourselves. However, when unexpected challenges are introduced, it leaves us with less time to organize for the transition: e.g., differences between practicing basketball shots from a penalty line on one's own and meeting unexpected challenges during a basketball game; or the difference in expected and unexpected challenges when practicing boxing with a punch bag as opposed to an unpredictable opponent, and so on.

Initially, it is safer to practice the organization duration on one's own and then escalate it by introducing unexpected challenges with a training companion.

GRADING SUBSKILLS

Many of our activities, such as soccer, often contain subskills which can be graded individually, and staggered within the activity plan. We have to keep in mind that every team player has a dedicated, skill-specific role, such as striker, defender, or goalkeeper; hence, they are likely to benefit from role-related rehabilitation. Now, imagine that the person with the lower limb condition described above is also a soccer player. They have improved the shared daily activities but are looking to recover playing soccer. A place to start could be with grading "non-ball" activities such as running, followed by sprinting, and then by more complex and demanding activities such as sidestepping, and so on. Once the player is considered to be suitably recovered, ball-related activities can be reintroduced in a graded manner. One possible start is to walk and gently dribble the ball. In the early stages, this could be even practiced at home while walking between rooms (this is, partly, a reassurance ploy). Force and velocity can be challenged by increasing the speed to gentle jogging and running with the ball, endurance by longer exposure, and movement range by increasing the step length (see Table 9.1). This can be followed by kicking the ball against the wall in the manner described above for the tennis serve: distance for force and velocity, repetition for endurance, and range of movement by short and long kicks from different positions or angles. This should be practiced with both affected and unaffected sides in order to challenge single-leg steadiness and balance (see below). This component can be further challenged by passing the ball from the inner to the outer step of the foot with the unaffected leg, while balancing on the affected side. Preferably, these activities should be practiced on the field for contextual effects (you learn specifically in the environment in which you practice, or you perform best in the environment in which you have practiced).

Activities such as dancing, which contain complex movement sequences, can also be graded within task. One possible approach is to have the dancer select the first minute from their current routine, but attenuate all the task parameters: use narrower movement ranges and less force, and slow down the sequence to a safe level. The parameters of that particular sequence can then be gradually amplified by adding other elements from the dance routine sequentially.

From the above, a general grading pattern emerges. In musculoskeletal conditions the remedial focus is directed at the task parameters; these components are challenged within the affected task(s). They are attenuated during the acute protection phase, whereas they are amplified during the restorative phase.

PROGRESSIVE AND REGRESSIVE MANAGEMENT

A patient has arrived in the clinic, complaining of reduced range of movement (ROM) or weakness of the hip due to a long-term injury. They have driven to the clinic and walked in, perhaps having to deal with a few steps on the way. At which level do we start the exercise management? Is there any point regressing them to activities that will provide a lower physical challenge, such as leg bench-presses performed sitting or recumbent, or exercise on the floor?

Ideally, a patient should exercise within their current movement capacity or above it. There is no therapeutic value in challenging movement at a level below the person's capacity. For example, rehabilitation of the hip, described above, would be in weight-bearing activities. Exercises on the floor or treatment table would be regressive, "sub-functional" challenges that are below the patient's capacity, and hence unlikely to offer any additional benefits.

Here are two progressive management considerations:

- Exclude extra-functional exercise if the patient is able to perform functional tasks.
- Exclude movement fragmentation if the patient is able to perform the whole task.

Is there a place for regressive management? It is reasoned that it is easier to train in a recumbent position or to fragment movement and then transfer this experience to functional tasks. However, these training/rehabilitation approaches are in conflict with specificity and motor control principles and are therefore unlikely to be effective (see Chapter 7). There are situations that require the movement challenges to be set at a level below the functional repertoire, especially in lower extremity conditions where body weight has to be partially eliminated, e.g., following Achilles tendon surgery. Under these circumstances, the use of regressive extra-functional challenges may be inevitable.

Another common argument for regressive management is that it may help reassure the patient that movement is safe. There may be some merit in this form of reassurance. For example, a person who had knee surgery may worry about weight-bearing activities (although they have walked into your clinic). To reassure them that movement is safe, the regressive management could for example commence with a recumbent cycling exercise. However, a regressive approach can also convey the opposite message: that functional movement is unsafe. If regressive reassurance is used, it should be swiftly replaced by functional challenges, preferably in the first session. For example, a patient who has come out of a leg plaster cast and is fearful about weight-bearing activities can be reassured by performing several off-weight-bearing "test" activities, such as dynamic and static leg exercises on the floor or treatment table (behavioral reassurance, Chapter 13). After a few cycles, I would remark on how well and "uneventful" these challenges were, highlighting that it is now safe to progress to the standing activities (cognitive reassurance, Chapter 13). However, when possible, it is preferable for the reassurance to commence with non-regressive functional activities, e.g., standing challenges.

DIRECTION OF ACTIVITY GRADING

The direction of grading can change in different conditions:

1) In all conditions associated with early phases of repair. Grading direction: initially attenuation of the task. Later, amplification toward the functional goal level.

2) In long-term conditions where physical capacity has been affected, such as following immobilization, detraining and neglect, in both musculoskeletal and CNS conditions. Direction of grading: from current level and amplified toward the functional goal.

3) In reassuring the patient that movement is safe (such as in chronic pain) and to increase engagement in individuals who withdraw from physical activities. Ideally, start grading from the current level and then amplify towards the functional goals. Occasionally, consider grading consisting of a brief (few minutes) attenuation in clinic followed immediately by amplification towards the functional goals.

> Activity grading using attenuation as an overall management should not to be used to alleviate persistent pain – it doesn't seem to work and may even reduce physical engagement (see Chapter 13). So, attenuation is used when there is acute injury or suspected damage. In most of the other musculoskeletal and pain conditions the direction of grading is from the current level and up towards the goal activity.

THE END-POINT OF GRADING AND TREATMENT?

In the best-case scenario, activity grading is terminated once the patient has reached their expressed goal of rehabilitation. This point is often represented by restoration of functionality to pre-injury/condition levels, or thereabouts. In a less favorable outcome, the grading ends when there is a clear plateau in improvement, which may be below the patient's desired outcome (see functional recovery and management goals, Chapter 2).

SUMMARY

- Activity grading is all about easing ourselves back to activity.

- Grading involves a stepwise increase or decrease in the intensity, demands, or complexity placed on an activity.

- During the protective phase of recovery, grading is in the direction of attenuation.

- During the restoration phase of recovery, grading is in the direction of amplification – avoid regressive activities/exercise.

- Both the whole task and its components can be graded.

- Component grading should be within the affected tasks.

- The patient should be involved in planning the grading program by defining their recovery goals and the scheduling particulars.

- Grading is terminated when the patient has achieved their target functionality, or when progress has reached a plateau.

In this part of the book you will explore how to construct an exercise management plan for acute and chronic pain and stiffness conditions:

All persistent pain, discomfort, and stiffness experiences
- Chronic low back and neck pain
- Chronic arthritic pain
- And possibly managing chronic tendinopathies and overuse injuries

Part 4
Supporting symptomatic alleviation

Chapter 10

Contents
Symptomatic recovery

To revisit the process approach model, it was proposed that in most musculoskeletal and pain conditions recovery is likely to take place through three key processes: repair (see Chapter 4), adaptation (see Chapter 6), and alleviation or modulation of symptoms, which is explored in the next three chapters (Fig. 10.1). We are now looking at the possibility of helping people recover their functionality but without necessarily providing a cure or inducing a physical change in their body. If you are not entirely convinced, consider what happens with placebos.

The focus in this part of the book will be on pain and stiffness, the two most common presenting symptoms in musculoskeletal practice. There is a deluge of research about pain but only a few drops in the way of stiffness, although in my clinical experience it may be as prevalent as pain presentations.

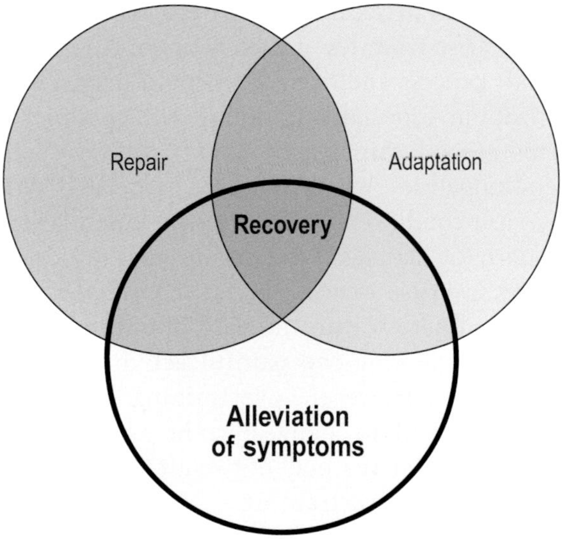

This section will explore the management of musculoskeletal pain conditions related to localized pain experiences rather than whole-body pain syndromes. Outside the scope of this book are pain conditions associated with systemic pathologies, such as autoimmune conditions or diabetic neuropathies; serious pathologies, such as cancer; and other complex pain conditions, such as regional pain syndromes and fibromyalgia.

PAIN PRESENTATIONS

As with medication, exercise prescription has, first and foremost, to be safe, but also must have the potency to alleviate symptoms. With this in mind and in the spirit of minimizing management complexity, pain conditions are divided here into two loose groups – *pain of injury* and *pain of sensitization* (or the more clinically communicative *pain of sensitivity*).

Injury-related pain presentations are associated with recent musculoskeletal tissue damage and the presence of an active repair process: i.e., all acute injuries and post-surgery conditions. Additionally, included in this group are overuse injuries, which are also associated with repair but often lack a clear onset and tend to persist beyond the expected duration of acute injuries. Another pain condition included in this group is the pain of delayed-onset muscle soreness (DOMS). It is associated with disruption to the sarcomeres' architecture but not necessarily with damage to or tears of the muscle fibers.

Pain of sensitivity represents conditions that are maintained beyond the expected duration of repair: *they are not* necessarily marked by

FIGURE 10.1
This part of the book explores functional recovery through alleviation of symptoms.

a repair process and may even be present in fully repaired tissues. Pain of sensitivity can be of any duration but is often associated with chronic pain, particularly if symptoms persist for 3–6 months after onset of the condition.[1] The terms "chronic pain" and "persistent pain" will be used interchangeably throughout this part of the book to imply pain of sensitization rather than injury.

Pain of fatigue and exertion is also considered within the sensitization group. These pain experiences are not associated with tissue damage. Injury-free individuals experience these activity-related symptoms; however, those suffering from sensitization tend to experience them more acutely and disproportionately to the activity.

PAIN OF INJURY

Pain that is the result of injury plays an essential protective role, providing the feedback needed for the individual to organize their actions to support tissue repair. This is exemplified by the commonly observed antalgic movement behavior – the limping in leg injuries and the functional scoliosis and stooping seen in acute back pain sufferers. This form of pain is expected to follow the course of repair, featuring prominently during the inflammatory phase and gradually diminishing as the inflammation and proliferation phases wind down. In mild injuries, this symptomatic improvement is likely to complete within 1–4 weeks, but it can extend up to several months in more severe conditions, such as nerve root compression by disk pathologies (see Chapter 4 for more on tissue damage).

Pain in overuse conditions

Overuse injuries are another group of conditions believed to be associated with tissue damage and marked by persistent pain and declining performance. They are described as injuries that result from repetitive stresses, progressing over time, and which do not have a distinct onset incident.[2] Overuse conditions are prevalent in sports.[3–5] They are predominantly seen in sports that involve long duration and repetitive training, such as cycling, swimming, long-distance running, throwing, and jumping. A prospective study of injuries among 313 athletes from different sports recorded 419 overuse problems in the knees, lower back, and shoulders during a 3-month period.[6] Of these, 34% were classified as substantial overuse problems, resulting in moderate to severe reductions in sports activities.

The presence of pain and loss of functionality is believed to be related to recurrent, ongoing, or incomplete tissue repair. These processes can be observed in all musculoskeletal structures, ranging from muscle damage and tendinopathies to stress fractures and damage to the subchondral bone and articular cartilage in adolescents (osteochondritis dissecans).[5] The persistence of pain could arise from the presence of an unresolved repair process and/or an element of neural sensitization, especially in long-term conditions. This central pain phenomenon is observed in tendinopathies, which are often associated with overuse conditions.[7–11] Due to the potential for underlying damage, and erring on the side of safety, overuse conditions are considered and managed here within the pain of injury group. Here, attenuating the painful activities seems reasonable. However, overtraining behaviors can be difficult to change,[12] as the psychological and social benefits may outweigh the pain and health costs of overtraining.

Pain of delayed-onset muscle soreness (DOMS)

Delayed muscle soreness is often experienced following a bout of unaccustomed exercise. It is marked by temporary muscle soreness, weakness, stiffness, and reduced range of movement.[13] The symptoms are short-lasting and tend to disappear within a few days to a week. Commonly in DOMS, the muscle fibers remain intact and whole. The damage is mostly restricted to sarcomeres in the form of shearing and disarrangement of the Z-bands and contractile mechanism (sometimes termed "sarcomere popping").

DOMS is a fast adaptation of muscle to exercise – a reorganization of the contractile apparatus to support the demands of the new activity. It is a rapid and highly effective process that tends to run its course within a few days to a week. By that time, the muscle is better adapted and resistant to DOMS from that particular activity.[13]

The disruption to the sarcomere is usually specific to selected myofibrils. The overall structure of the muscle and fascia remains intact and therefore the tensile strength is unlikely to be compromised.[14] Hence, it is safe to continue training while experiencing DOMS, but it can be a somewhat unpleasant experience.

PAIN OF SENSITIZATION

Pain of sensitization is somewhat of an enigma. It seems that we can suffer from a pain condition without having underlying tissue damage or ongoing repair. Persistent musculoskeletal pain beyond 3–6 months is considered to be related to persistent sensitization: a pain condition which is maintained by central neurological processes rather than peripheral tissue damage. These pain disorders are prevalent and are commonly seen in chronic conditions such as low back and neck pain, tendinopathies,[7] tension headaches, and symptomatic osteoarthritis. Clinically, a person is considered to be within the sensitization group if they present with persistent musculoskeletal pain which is experienced well beyond the expected duration of repair. Excluded from this group are persistent unresolved chronic inflammatory conditions, such as autoimmune disorders.

To understand how the pain experience can become persistent, we need to look at the biological role of sensitization. Following injury, sensitization plays an important protective role during repair; it lets us know that we have sustained tissue damage. This happens by lowering of the nociceptors' thresholds at the site of damage, combined with a lowering of synaptic thresholds along central nociceptive pathways (Fig. 10.2).[15] Tissue injury initiates a frenzy of chemical communication between all the cells at the site of damage, including the damaged cells, vascular, immune, and repair cells, and local nociceptors. The presence of these molecules excites the nociceptors and lowers their activation threshold. In turn, the activated nociceptors release various neurotransmitters from their terminals (such as substance P), which induce vasodilatation and further stimulate the local immune cells. Now everything is really excited! In essence, sensitization sharpens the detection of noxious events and facilitates the transmission of this information centrally.

The lowering of thresholds of the nociceptors and central pathways gives rise to heightened sensitivity to stimuli that do not normally elicit pain, such as movement of joints and muscle activity. This central hypersensitivity tends to spread and affect the surrounding undamaged tissues.[16] A person with a low back injury might experience pain and stiffness in their hamstrings when bending forward, although these tissues are undamaged. They often experience diffuse hypersensitivity when pressure is applied by palpation to the iliac crest, iliotibial tract,

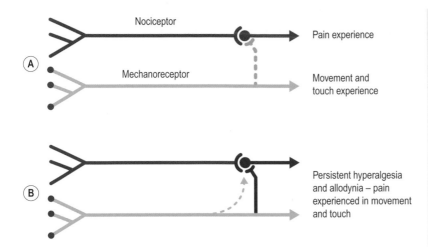

Nociceptor

Pain experience

(A)

Mechanoreceptor

Movement and
touch experience

(B)

Persistent hyperalgesia
and allodynia – pain
experienced in movement
and touch

FIGURE 10.2
(A) Normal sensation.
Nociceptive and
mechanoreceptive signals
are transmitted via distinct
pathways. (B) Persistent
sensitization: a state of
sensitization remains,
although the repair process
has been completed. It should
be noted that sensitization is a
whole nervous system/person
phenomenon and this is one
element within this process.
(*Allodynia*: the experience of
pain from stimuli that is not
normally painful. *Hyperalgesia*:
abnormally increased
sensitivity to painful stimuli.)

and gluteal areas, although these structures are somewhat distant from where the injury is expected to be. This can give rise to false-positive findings that result in unnecessary hamstring stretches or deep massage of these sensitive yet undamaged structures (Chapter 12; see being stiff versus feeling stiff). From a protective perspective, this spread of sensitivity probably serves to inform us that we are getting closer to the area of damage, a bit like the "hot and cold" children's game.

With most injuries, sensitization tends to diminish and eventually disappear in line with the resolution of repair. However, substantial numbers of people with acute musculoskeletal pain go on to develop chronic pain that persists long after tissue healing has taken place.[17] For example, a year after an acute neck or low back episode, 22–30% of individuals still experience some level of pain.[17–19] In these conditions, *the generator of pain is no longer associated with*

tissue damage and repair but with a persistent version of the sensitization seen in acute injury (Fig. 10.3), i.e., ongoing peripheral and central change in thresholds. Sensitization's longevity may be related to neuroplasticity within the pain-experiencing system where "neurons wire together if they fire together" (Hebb's rule). This means that the pain pathways become more efficient with recurrent and prolonged pain experiences.[16] We know that the central nervous system has the capacity to form such long-term pain memories that outlast injury. This is seen in phantom limb pain, where a person can re-experience the pain of an old injury which occurred many years before the limb was amputated.

Persistent sensitization is often considered to be an accompanying symptom of other ailments; however, it is a separate condition in its own right.[20] It has no obvious biological protective role and is probably a disorder

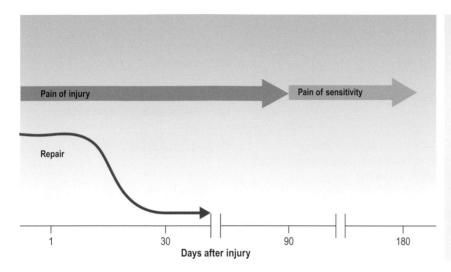

FIGURE 10.3
Pain of injury and sensitivity. Pain experienced beyond the period of repair (3–6 months) is likely to be generated by central nervous system processes.

affecting the "pain-experiencing system." It is well documented that biopsychosocial and environmental factors affect the course of sensitization. Familial factors, such as parental chronic pain, are associated with chronic non-specific multisite pain in adolescents and young adults.[21] Some 50% of chronic pain conditions can be attributed to genetics.[22] It can occur as a sequela to severe physical trauma or surgery, but then most of the patients that I see have no recollection of how it came about; one day, a long time ago, it was just there. Psychological factors, such as trauma and depression, are often stated as a contributing factor,[18] yet in clinic I frequently see happy people who are very unhappy about their ongoing pain. By the very nature of the pain being chronic, a patient with sensitization will seek help weeks or months after the condition started. With the passage of time, it can be difficult to unpick the factors that gave rise to their condition. Hence, removing the causes and the maintaining factors of sensitization can be challenging in clinic.

Some differences between pain of injury and sensitization are shown in Table 10.1.

A note on the use of the term "chronic" in clinic: various chronic conditions can potentially resolve many months after their onset. This is seen in conditions such as frozen shoulder, back and neck pain, and tendinopathies.[18,23–26] However, the term chronic pain could be interpreted by the patient as being irrevocable pain. They are more likely to describe their symptoms and the length of time they have experienced them, and rarely label their persistent condition as being chronic. Perhaps using alternative terms such as "remaining/residual/lasting sensitivity" would be more beneficial to describe the condition and prepare the individual for management which aims, in part, to reduce this sensitivity.

Pain of fatigue and exertion

A common clinical presentation is a person who suffers from low back pain which is made worse by prolonged standing or walking. Often, this pain is alleviated when they take a few minutes' rest, after which they can often resume that activity. So, we are now looking at the pain of doing too much – the pain of fatigue and exertion.

Table 10.1 Some clinical features of pain of injury and sensitization

	Pain of injury	Pain of sensitivity
Onset	History of trauma	Often unknown cause Can develop following physical trauma/ops
Duration	Any pain within 3 months of injury (many injuries likely to recover symptomatically well within 3–8 weeks)	Ongoing pain over 3–6 months
Movement behavior	Protective movement strategies Antalgic postures/gait	Movement fears Absence of protective movement strategies
Symptomatic area	Local related to area of damage Neurological symptoms along clear peripheral pathway	Diffuse non-anatomical Fleeting aches and pains, different areas Multiple sites of persistent/recurrent pain
Pattern	Clear onset, a peak and gradual attenuation	Ongoing or intermittent, no clear pattern
Palpation	Hypersensitivity local to damaged tissues Focal area of pain	Wide area of allodynia and hypersensitivity Tender points in remote areas from the site of primary pain

Fatigue is experienced during intense exercise as loss of force production and pain, often described as "the burn" in sports.[27] The physiological role of these sensations is to provide protection from the harmful effects of over-exercising.[28] Importantly, fatigue is not associated with deleterious effect on tissues; it seems to kick in long before tissue or system damage occurs.

In some circumstances, especially in persistent conditions, the pain of fatigue can be experienced as being harmful.[29] For example, when subjects with chronic trapezius pain and asymptomatic controls were given a repetitive task of moving a light object between two positions, they both experienced the pain of fatigue.[30] The pain-free group experienced a mild discomfort, which recovered soon after the task was terminated. In comparison, the symptomatic group started off at a higher pain level, spiking dramatically during the exercise period and taking longer to recover to their baseline pain level. In this study, the pain experienced by the symptomatic group reached a level of 70 mm on a 100 mm visual analog scale (VAS, Fig. 10.4). For most individuals, this pain level would equate with a substantial injury. Although the pain can be intense, if we were to peer into the symptomatic muscle, we would not observe any signs of

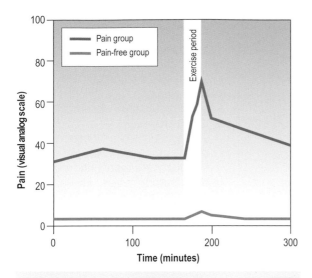

FIGURE 10.4

Sensitization and pain of fatigue in individuals with chronic trapezius pain. Both pain and pain-free groups experience the pain of fatigue during a light repetitive task. However, the pain group starts off with a higher level of pain, which spikes during performance of the task. (After Rosendal L, Larsson B, Kristiansen J, Peolsson M, Søgaard K, Kjær M, et al. Increase in muscle nociceptive substances and anaerobic metabolism in patients with trapezius myalgia: microdialysis in rest and during exercise. Pain. 2004;112:324–34.)

tissue damage or active repair process. It seems to be orchestrated within the physiological and neural dimensions, probably by the neurogenic sensitization described above.

The experience of pain during exertion is another enigma yet to be illuminated. For example, in a group of healthy individuals given a prolonged task, such as standing for over 45 minutes, some 70% of the subjects will develop some form of leg and/or low back pain (Fig. 10.5).[31] However, this pain tends to fade

away once the task is terminated.[32] If this study is repeated with a group of individuals who suffer from ongoing low back pain, they will experience the same pattern of pain, except that it will be more intense.[33] They, too, will recover to their default pain level at the end of the task, suggesting that the pain of exertion is not associated with tissue damage but a benign, centralized, and transient pain phenomenon.

During prolonged and sustained physical activities, we all experience some form of discomfort associated with fatigue and exertion, but individuals who are already sensitized feel it a lot more and for longer. During a long walk, sitting at work, or standing in a queue we may all experience some mild low back discomfort related to fatigue or exertion. However, a person with chronic pain will experience it more intensely. Often, this experience is mixed with unfounded fears that the pain represents progressive tissue damage. Consequently, they may self-limit or withdraw from activities that are otherwise safe and beneficial. This has important implications for exercise prescription for individuals suffering from chronic pain. They may experience the transient pain of fatigue and exertion during the exercise, which they may erroneously associate with injury or a worsening condition. This can be overcome by explaining the transient and unharmful nature of the pain of fatigue and exertion and the benefits of maintaining physical activity for overall pain management and health (see cognitive and behavioral reassurance, Chapter 13).

Research has looked at an array of possible causes for the pain of exertion, from blood pooling, ligamentous creep, and motor control issues to postural factors.[31] In chronic low back conditions, no correlation was found between any of these factors and developing pain, except for

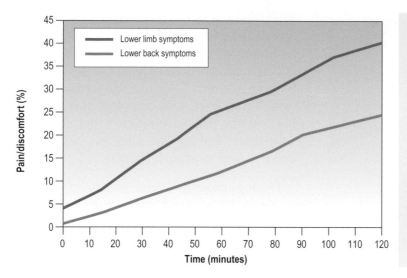

FIGURE 10.5
Pooled dose–response association between prolonged standing (in minutes) and low back symptoms and lower limb symptoms (pain or discomfort, on a 0–100 scale). (After Coenen P. Associations of prolonged standing with musculoskeletal symptoms – a systematic review of laboratory studies. Gait Posture. 2017;58:310–18.)

prolonged standing in a stooped position and marked lumbar lordosis.[33,34] So, from a management point of view, introducing breaks or changes in activities seems to be a reasonable solution. But then, these benign aches and pains are not associated with developing tissue damage. So, depending on the circumstances, another option is to persevere in spite of pain. The worst that could happen is a transient increase in pain. However, we have to be mindful of the overuse conditions seen in athletes, where persistent pain may be associated with tissue damage.

Sensitization: biopsychosocial not biomechanical

The cause, persistence, and resolution of sensitization occur within the biopsychosocial sphere rather than a structural dimension. A biopsychosocial model is inclusive of biological processes, psychological, environmental, and social influences, whereas the biomechanical dimension refers to musculoskeletal structure, posture biomechanics, and physical capacity (strength, endurance, and flexibility). Chronic pain has been shown consistently to be associated with biopsychosocial factors but rarely with biomechanical factors such as poor posture or bending techniques, joint flexibility, or muscle imbalances.[35–39] Despite these findings, strength, endurance, and flexibility exercises are still the most popular modalities used in the management of chronic pain – and they can be effective, up to a point (see Chapter 11). Strength training is one of the most prescribed exercises for managing pain, on the widely held belief that a "strong body knows no pain." However, low physical capacity is not seen as a risk factor for developing low back, neck, and shoulder pain.[40–41] A person with high physical capacity is just as likely to experience pain as a person with low capacity.[40–41] Ironically, athletes who are likely to have a higher than normal physical capacity often suffer from a multitude of acute and persistent pain conditions.[6,42–44]

Although biomechanical factors are not believed to be the cause of chronic pain, paradoxically, symptoms can be alleviated by exercise which *seems* to target biomechanical anomalies:

for example, quadriceps-strengthening exercises to alleviate osteoarthritic knee pain or core exercise to reduce spinal pain. This inconsistency can be resolved by recognizing that all exercises modulate chronic pain and that this effect is mediated within the biopsychosocial dimension. Hence, all exercises seem to "work" but their effects are unrelated to physical changes within the musculoskeletal system (see Chapter 11).

SAFETY OF EXERCISING WHILE IN PAIN

Generally, a person recovering from most musculoskeletal and pain conditions is better off with some form of activity than not. It is more about setting a safe activity level. In respect to the two pain groups (pain of injury and pain of sensitivity), safety concerns are mainly related to the pain of injury where there is damage and reduced tissue tensile strength. In pain sensitivity conditions, the symptomatic area is likely to be intact and possess the same tensile properties as similar asymptomatic tissues. Hence, early unattenuated return to activity may reinjure a recently damaged tissue but "only" worsen the symptoms in pain sensitivity conditions.

In acute injuries, hurt is associated with harm and activities should be attenuated accordingly. Estimated minor damage can be managed by attenuating the task parameters within the shared repertoire (e.g., short walks), whereas extensive injuries may need more dramatic decrease in loading to a sub-functional level (e.g., off-weight-bearing activities). The activity progression in severe injury could be from extra-functional to attenuated daily activities, then amplified daily activity, and, eventually, a gradual return to the unique repertoire, such as the principal sporting activity. Regardless of the form of exercise or extent of damage, the remedial movement should initially be within comfortable and tolerable intensity and ranges: a "let pain guide you" approach. However, this advice is not without its limitations. The intensity of pain does not always reflect the magnitude of underlying damage.

The issue of pain and safety is different in chronic pain conditions. Persistent sensitization has an elusive biological role. It does not seem to provide any protective function, as would the pain of injury. The repair process is expected to resolve well before the 3–6 months' duration associated with chronicity.[1] Hence, individuals who have persistent pain do not necessarily have underlying damage or "weaker tissues" that would make them more susceptible to injury.[1] There is nothing to protect in sensitization except the state of being in pain itself. Pain in sensitization is hurt but not harm. Hence, a person experiencing sensitivity is as safe to exercise as an asymptomatic one.

The message that hurt is not harm extends to the pain of fatigue and exertion. Under normal circumstances, these two phenomena are likely to be a biological safety valve to prevent overuse injury and systemic failure. However, they both seem to kick in long before tissue failure – but more intensely so in a sensitized individual. In the pain of fatigue and exertion, the underlying tissues are likely to be intact and possess the tensile strength of similar non-sensitive tissues. Hence, it is reasonably safe to persevere with activities and, if necessary, introduce a short rest.

From an activity-grading perspective, in acute conditions first attenuate the activity level and then progressively amplify it using the grading approach described in Chapter 9. In chronic pain which is not associated with tissue damage, the person can be encouraged to maintain or even increase their physical engagement, particularly if they have withdrawn from exercise or physical activities due to persistent pain. Research suggests that chronic pain sufferers who set their goal to preserve their functional repertoire tend to have better outcomes in terms of symptoms, functionality, and well-being.[45–47]

repair. Pain of sensitivity is due to residual neural sensitivity, possibly related to a past injury. It is not associated with tissue damage or weakness." This is usually followed by safety reassurance messages, for example:

How to explain the pain of sensitivity: "There are two types of pain conditions: pain of injury and pain of sensitivity. Pain of injury is acute and short-lasting, and is associated with injury and

"Your painful back is as strong as that of a person without pain – it's just more sensitive", "Your painful Achilles is as strong as the tendon on the other side – it's just more sensitive," and so on.

Follow this with a call for action:

"We need to find a way to reduce this sensitivity; exercise can be one of them."

SUMMARY

- Pain conditions can be divided into two broad groups – pain of injury and pain of sensitivity.
- Pain of injury includes damage brought about by acute strains, blunt trauma, DOMS, and overuse injuries.
- Pain of sensitivity is associated with pain conditions that persist 3–6 months beyond onset.
- Pain of injury is associated with tissue damage and repair.
- Persistent pain is a central nervous system, biological, whole-person process.
- Persistent pain is unrelated to tissue damage, biomechanics, posture, or motor control issues.
- Individuals who suffer from persistent pain and who are already sensitive may experience greater pain during fatigue and exertion.
- In persistent pain conditions, exercise prescription should target the central, whole-person processes – there may be nothing to put right in the periphery.

References

1. Treede RD, Rief W, Barke A, Aziz Q, Bennett MI, Benoliel R, et al. A classification of chronic pain for ICD-11. Pain. 2015;156:1003–7.

2. Bahr R. No injuries, but plenty of pain? On the methodology for recording overuse symptoms in sports. Br J Sports Med. 2009;43:966–72.

3. Myklebust G, Hasslan L, Bahr R, Steffen K. High prevalence of shoulder pain among elite Norwegian female handball players. Scand J Med Sci Sports. 2013;23:288–94.

4. van Beijsterveldt AM, Richardson A, Clarsen B, Stubbe J. Sports injuries and illnesses in first-year physical education teacher education students. BMJ Open Sport Exerc Med. 2017;3:e000189.

5. Aicale R, Tarantino D, Maffulli N. Overuse injuries in sport: a comprehensive overview. J Orthop Surg Res. 2018;13:309.

6. Clarsen B, Myklebust G, Bahr R. Development and validation of a new method for the registration of overuse injuries in sports injury epidemiology: the Oslo Sports Trauma Research Centre (OSTRC) Overuse Injury Questionnaire. Br J Sports Med. 2013;47:495–502.

7. Färnqvist K. Treating tendinopathies – are we searching for a needle in a haystack, when we should include the whole haystack? Eur J Physiother. 2020;23:63–5.

8. de Jonge S, Tol JL, Weir A, Waarsing JH, Verhaar JAN, de Vos R-J. The tendon structure returns to asymptomatic values in nonoperatively treated Achilles tendinopathy but is not associated with symptoms: a prospective study. Am J Sports Med. 2015;43:2950–8.

9. Alfredson H, Lorentzon R. Chronic tendon pain: no signs of chemical inflammation but high concentrations of the neurotransmitter glutamate. Implications for treatment? Curr Drug Targets. 2002;31:43–54.

10. Scott A, Bahr R. Neuropeptides in tendinopathy. Front Biosci. 2009;14:2203–11.

11. Andersson G, Danielson P, Alfredson H, Forsgren S. Presence of substance P and the neurokinin-1 receptor in tenocytes of the human Achilles tendon. Regul Pept. 2008;150:81–7.

12. Andrews NE, Strong J, Meredith PJ, Gordon K, Bagraith KS. "It's very hard to change yourself": an exploration of overactivity in people with chronic pain using interpretative phenomenological analysis. Pain. 2015;156:1215–31.

13. Hortobágyi T, Houmard J, Fraser D, Dudek R, Lambert J, Tracy J. Normal forces and myofibrillar disruption after repeated eccentric exercise. J Appl Physiol. 1998;84:492–8.

14. Fridén J, Sjöström M, Ekblom B. Myofibrillar damage following intense eccentric exercise in man. Int J Sports Med. 1983;4:170-6.

15. Garland EL. Pain processing in the human nervous system: a selective review of nociceptive and biobehavioral pathways. Prim Care. 2012;39:561–71.

16. Woolf CJ. Central sensitization: implications for the diagnosis and treatment of pain. Pain. 2011;152:S2–S15.

17. Kasch H, Qerama E, Kongsted A, Bach FW, Bendix T, Jensen TS. Deep muscle pain, tender points and recovery in acute whiplash patients: a 1-year follow-up study Pain. 2008;140:65–73.

18. Henschke N, Maher CG, Refshauge KM, et al. Prognosis in patients with recent onset low back pain in Australian primary care: inception cohort study. BMJ. 2008;337:a171.

19. Itz CJ, Geurts JW, van Kleef M, Nelemans P. Clinical course of non-specific low back pain: a systematic review of prospective cohort studies set in primary care. Eur J Pain. 2013;17:5–15.

20. Mills SEE, Nicolson KP, Smith BH. Chronic pain: a review of its epidemiology and associated factors in population-based studies. Br J Anaesth. 2019;123:e273–e283.

21. Hoftun GB, Romundstad PR, Rygg M. Association of parental chronic pain with chronic pain in the adolescent and young adult: family linkage data from the HUNT Study. JAMA Pediatr. 2013;167:61–9.

22. Stone AL, Wilson AC. Transmission of risk from parents with chronic pain to offspring. Pain. 2016;157:2628–39.

23. Shaffer B, Tibone JE, Kerlan RK. Frozen shoulder. A long-term follow-up. J Bone Joint Surg Am. 1992;74:738–46.

24. Hand C, Clipsham K, Rees JL, Carr AJ. Long-term outcome of frozen shoulder. J Shoulder Elbow Surg. 2008;17:231–6.

25. Ferrari R. Prevention of chronic pain after whiplash. Emerg Med J. 2002;19:526–30.

26. Bisset L, Beller E, Jull G, Brooks P, Darnell R, Vicenzino B. Mobilization with movement and exercise, corticosteroid injection, or wait and see for tennis elbow: randomised trial. BMJ. 2006;333:939.

27. Pollak KA, Swenson JD, Vanhaitsma TA, Hughen RW, Jo D, White AT, et al. Exogenously applied muscle metabolites synergistically evoke sensations of muscle fatigue and pain in human subjects. Exp Physiol. 2014;99:368–80.

28. Ament W, Verkerke GJ. Exercise and fatigue. Sports Med. 2009;39:389–422.

29. Lima LV, Abner TSS, Sluka KA. Does exercise increase or decrease pain? Central mechanisms underlying these two phenomena. J Physiol. 2017;595: 4141–50.

30. Rosendal L, Larsson B, Kristiansen J, Peolsson M, Søgaard K, Kjær M, et al. Increase in muscle nociceptive substances and anaerobic metabolism in patients with trapezius myalgia: microdialysis in rest and during exercise. Pain. 2004;112:324–34.

31. Coenen P. Associations of prolonged standing with musculoskeletal symptoms: a systematic review of laboratory studies. Gait Posture. 2017;58:310–18.

32. Gallagher KM, Callaghan JP. Early static standing is associated with prolonged standing induced low back pain. Hum Mov Sci. 2015;44:111–21.

33. Sorensen CJ, Johnson MB, Callaghan JP, George SZ, Van Dillen LR. Validity of a paradigm for low back pain symptom development during prolonged standing. Clin J Pain. 2015;31:652–9.

34. Gregory DE, Callaghan JP. Prolonged standing as a precursor for the development of low back discomfort: an investigation of possible mechanisms. Gait Posture. 2008;28:86–92.

35. Parreira P, Maher CG, Steffens D, Hancock MJ, Ferreira ML. Risk factors for low back pain and sciatica: an umbrella review. Spine J. 2018;18:1715–21.

36. McLean SM, May S, Klaber-Moffett J, Sharp DM, Gardiner E. Risk factors for the onset of nonspecific neck pain: a systematic review. J Epidemiol Community Health. 2010;64:565–72.

37. Nijs J, Roussel N, Paul van Wilgen C, Köke A, Smeets R. Thinking beyond muscles and joints: therapists' and patients' attitudes and beliefs regarding chronic musculoskeletal pain are key to applying effective treatment. Man Ther. 2013;18:96–102.

38. Lederman E. The myth of core stability. J Bodyw Mov Ther. 2010;14:84–98.

39. Lederman E. The fall of the postural-structural-biomechanical model in manual and physical therapies: exemplified by lower back pain. J Bodyw Mov Ther. 2011;15:131–8.

40. Hamberg-van Reenen HH, Ariëns GAM, Blatter BM, van der Beek AJ, Twisk JWR, van Mechelen W, et al. Is an imbalance between physical capacity and exposure to work-related physical factors associated with low-back, neck or shoulder pain? Scand J Work Environ Health. 2006;32:190–7.

41. Hamberg-van Reenen HH, Ariëns GA, Blatter BM, van Mechelen W, Bongers PM. A systematic review of the relation between physical capacity and future low back and neck/shoulder pain. Pain. 2007;130:93–107.

42. Trompeter K, Fett D, Platen P. Prevalence of back pain in sports: a systematic review of the literature. Sports Med. 2017;47:1183–207.

43. Noormohammadpour P, Farahbakhsh F, Farahbakhsh F, Rostami M, Kordi R. Prevalence of neck pain among athletes: a systematic review. Asian Spine J. 2018;12:1146–53.

44. Hainline B, Derman W, Vernec A, Budgett R, Deie M, Dvořák J, et al. International Olympic Committee consensus statement on pain management in elite athletes. Br J Sports Med. 2017;51:1245–58.

45. Zale EL, Lange KL, Fields SA, Ditre JW. The relation between pain-related fear and disability: a meta-analysis. J Pain. 2013;14: 1019–30.

46. Kindermans HP, Roelofs J, Goossens ME, Huijnen IP, Verbunt JA, Vlaeyen JW. Activity patterns in chronic pain: underlying dimensions and associations with disability and depressed mood. J Pain. 2011;12:1049–58.

47. Andrews NE, Strong J, Meredith PJ. Activity pacing, avoidance, endurance, and associations with patient functioning in chronic pain: a systematic review and meta-analysis. Arch Phys Med Rehabil. 2012;93:2109–21.e7.

Chapter 11

Contents
Exercise and pain alleviation

Two patients suffering from low back pain: one suffering from acute pain, the other from ongoing discomfort and stiffness – both looking for pain alleviation through some form of remedial exercise. Which exercise or activity will be beneficial?

It is not uncommon for a patient who is experiencing pain to report that, while exercising – e.g., playing soccer or running – they are not aware of their condition. What is the process by which such pain alleviation occurs? Can we "bottle" it and apply it lavishly in the exercise plan?

SOURCE OF PAIN MODULATION

Imagine that you are hiking in some remote area and happen to trip and sprain your ankle. As you are sitting there, the pain increases and you find it difficult to get up and walk any distance. No one is around to help and your cabin is half an hour's walk away. As you contemplate your misfortune, a bear appears in the distance. Without a thought, you spring up and sprint, with the bear now in close pursuit. In the nick of time, you reach the cabin, stumble in, shut the door behind you, and slump on the sofa, exhausted. After a while, the ankle becomes very painful and swollen. With great effort, you manage to get up, limp to the fireplace, add a few logs, and then hobble back to the sofa and doze off. You suddenly awake with a start; the room is filled with smoke. While asleep, one of the logs rolled out of the fireplace, setting the cabin on fire. Without giving the injury a thought, you spring up and sprint out of the door to escape the raging inferno – only to find the bear waiting for you on the other side.

This melodrama may be a bit of a long story, but it aims to convey important principles that relate to exercise and modulation of symptoms. The pain experience is a potent behavior modifier, yet its intensity can be regulated according to prevailing circumstances.[1] In injury, pain serves as a feedback system that helps steer our defensive and protective actions, depending on current priorities. However, pain itself can be centrally modulated to support the execution of these movement strategies. Hence, it can be attenuated to enable escape behavior during emergencies (fight or flight).[2] When we are in a safe environment, pain sensitivity may rise to guide the protective movement behavior that supports damage limitation – the commonly observed antalgic posture and gait. Later in the repair process, there is a gradual lowering of sensitivity that enables the restorative behavior – the gradual loading of tissues in parallel with the return of tensile strength, the "baby steps" people take as they progressively resume their functional repertoire.

The pain experience "resides" within our nervous system and is therefore influenced by a wide array of psychological, behavioral, and social factors, as well as levels of physical activity or exercise. There are higher central nervous system (CNS)/brain functions and whole-person processes that regulate the pain experience through reflexive, non-conscious, and conscious processes (Fig. 11.1). The modulation of pain is then organized and transmitted via several central pathways and neurophysiological processes. These include the endogenous opioid and endocannabinoid systems, descending nociceptive inhibitory mechanisms, the hypothalamus–pituitary–adrenal axis, and the autonomic nervous system.[3-4] However, a recent

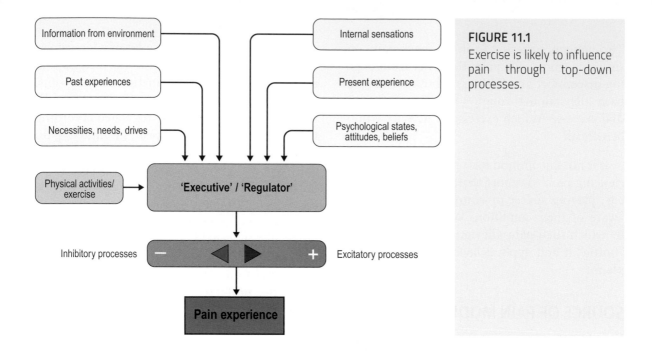

FIGURE 11.1
Exercise is likely to influence pain through top-down processes.

systematic review could not reach firm conclusions about the impact of exercise on the concentrations of pain-relieving peptides or their effects on areas linked to pain processing.[5]

Being active and exercising has many benefits that can influence these central processes and therefore the pain experience. Exercise can change the relationship of the individual to their pain experience by influencing psychological factors such as fear avoidance and catastrophizing. Exercises are all about self-care – they can re-establish a sense of control and install a feeling of optimism that improvement may be possible. This could explain why prescribed exercises are more effective in the short term. This may be due to their novelty value, which comes with a sense of control and hope but fades as the activity becomes habitual and wearisome. There is also the effect of activity on self-image and self-esteem. These psychological processes

outlast the duration of exercise, and are likely to confer long-term symptomatic improvements and contribute to the overall well-being of the individual.

Another potential candidate for exercise-induced pain modulation is related to attentional processes.[6] In essence, there is a hierarchy in attentional processes that tends to favor more salient events while filtering out less relevant information:[2] a sort of competition in attention.[7] Pain, having a protective function, often wins this competition, even in chronic conditions where it no longer serves this protective role.[8] However, the pain experience can be modulated according to the locus of attention. When attention is focused on pain, it is perceived as more intense, and less so when the focus is distracted away from it.[2] So, while reading this paragraph you might not be aware of the mild discomfort of sitting; but now that attention is drawn to it, you are more likely to feel it. Similarly, individuals who have chronic pain tend to overfocus internally on their symptom,[2] which is likely to intensify their pain experience. Exercise and activities that contain clear external goals that divert attention from the body may therefore contribute to pain attenuation.

Movement itself may have an immediate and transient modulating effect on pain related to spinal-level processing. In the 1960s, Melzack and Wall demonstrated that nociceptive transmission can be interrupted at a spinal cord level by concurrent mechanoreceptive stimulation (vibration).[9] This inhibitory process, too, is highly contextual, depending on the prevailing circumstances, as discussed above. It could explain the common observation that certain pain sufferers prefer some movement in the symptomatic area, usually in the form of cyclical and low-load activity. For example, individuals with low back pain often stand and rhythmically rock or walk as a way of controlling their symptoms. Also, during the painful phase of frozen shoulder, it was demonstrated that cyclical passive motion or low-force pendulum swings of the shoulder are effective in helping regulate pain (see Chapter 14 for a demonstration).[10] They are also useful after hip arthroscopy, but these benefits were related to repair quality rather than pain control (see Chapters 4 and 5).[11] Basically, more research is needed in this area.

There is a widely held belief in physical therapies and sports that a "strong body" or an "ideal body" knows no pain. In this bottom-up model, symptomatic improvements from exercise are often attributed to biomechanical modification, structural and postural repatterning, or improvements in movement capacity (strength, endurance, and flexibility). However, these approaches may be missing the important therapeutic target.

The development of and recovery from chronic musculoskeletal pain are largely associated with biopsychosocial rather than physical factors.[12] Persistent pain is generated and sustained by CNS processes. Exercise modulates the pain experience through these top-down central processes, such as their effects on mood, anxiety, sense of well-being, attentional processes, self- and body-image, and change in attitude and relationship of the individual to their pain.[13–14]

Pain modulation is a phenomenon that *may* occur during exercise; however, its direction and potency depend on an array of biopsychosocial factors, attitudes, beliefs and expectations, previous pain experiences, type of pain condition, intensity of exercise, and, to a lesser extent, the type of exercise prescribed.[4,15–16]

EXERCISE-INDUCED PAIN MODULATION

Exercise-induced pain modulation is described as the change in the experience of pain that occurs during and following exercise. The immediate effects of exercise are often evaluated by delivering a painful stimulus before, during, and after exercise, and measuring the changes in the person's perception of pain levels. In pain-free individuals, an intense bout of aerobic or resistance exercise has a predictable hypoalgesic effect on the induced pain that can last for up to 30 minutes.[3] The hypoalgesic effect tends to rise with the intensity of the exercise,[17,18] and painful exercise may bring about greater hypoalgesia than non-painful exercise.[15] Generally, either aerobic or resistance activities can bring about hypoalgesia with a moderate effect size in aerobic exercise and a large effect size in isometric and dynamic resistance exercise.[19]

Athletes who are "familiar" with pain during training or competitions, such as triathletes, exhibit greater pain tolerance and more efficient pain modulation than controls.[20,21] This may be mediated by psychological factors that enable better coping with fear of pain and mental stress.[20,21] Interestingly, placebo seems to produce an equal level of hypoalgesia as isotonic exercise, whereas nocebo can override and turn the exercise-induced hypoalgesia into hyperalgesia.[16] So, the brain and the person contribute a lot to pain modulation. Added to the complexity of exercise-induced hypoalgesia, and somewhat paradoxically, exercise itself can be painful and individuals can experience marked muscle pain during intensive training.[22]

The testing methods described above may not give a full picture of exercise-induced pain modulation. In these studies, pain is inflicted on asymptomatic individuals who have no underlying tissue damage or pre-existing neural sensitization. Unlike pain-free individuals, chronic pain sufferers may have a disorder in their pain-experiencing system.[23] When tested using the method above, their responses to exercise can be varied and somewhat unpredictable. Depending on the pain condition and the intensity of the workout, the inflicted pain can remain unchanged, reduce or worsen.[18–19]

Generally, hyperalgesic responses tend to occur more frequently in individuals with diffuse pain disorders, such as chronic whiplash disorder, fibromyalgia, and chronic fatigue syndrome. In contrast, patients with localized chronic conditions, such as shoulder myalgia, may experience hyperalgesia following isometric or repetitive movement of the local muscles; conversely, they experience hypoalgesia when contracting remote, non-affected muscles.[24] Similarly, people with painful osteoarthritis of the knee may experience hyperalgesia when performing resistance exercise in the painful lower limb, but a hypoalgesic response when exercising the upper limbs.[25]

Furthermore, the laboratory studies on exercise-induced hypoalgesia may not reflect what happens in the "real world" of remedial exercise. These studies suggest that more intense and painful training could lead to greater hypoalgesia. However, exercise such as tai chi, which is a low-intensity, low-impact, and largely pain-free practice, can alleviate chronic pain and improve function.[26–27] Additionally, there may be a "U-shaped" relationship between exercise and chronic pain, where a moderate volume of exercise reduces pain, but excessive training may increase it.[28,29] This U-shaped relationship has also been observed in recreational exercise and cardiovascular health, where excessive training negates the positive effect of moderate exercise.[30]

EXERCISE EFFECT ON CHRONIC MUSCULOSKELETAL PAIN AND FUNCTIONALITY

Of particular importance for constructing a remedial management plan are clinical studies that explore the long-term effects of exercise on persistent pain. On the whole, these studies demonstrate that all forms of exercise are beneficial for managing chronic pain.[31–34] Regular moderate recreational exercise 1–3 times per week is associated with a lower incidence of chronic pain in the general population, from a prevalence of 29% to approximately 19% in the exercising population.[28]

Generally, the effect size of all exercise on chronic pain conditions is small to medium and is most noticeable in the short term.[31,32] For example, exercise for osteoarthritis of the knee reduces pain by an average of 1.0 points on a 0–10 numerical scale and improves physical function by an average of 1.0 points.[35] In the arthritic hip, exercise reduces pain by 0.8 points and improves function by 0.7 points.[36] In chronic low back conditions, exercise improves pain by 0.7 points and function by 0.25 points in individuals from the general population. For those already attending a healthcare provider, the improvement was greater: 1.3 points for pain and 0.7 for function.[37] Short-term improvements in chronic neck pain follow a similar trend – approximately 1.5 points for pain and approximately 0.5 points for functionality. By 6 months of exercise, the effect seems to wear off to 1.0 points in pain alleviation. Pain modulation as a biopsychosocial phenomenon is not exclusive to exercise. Even clinical procedures such as history taking and physical examination reduce pain by 1.2 points in the low back and 0.95 points in the leg, as well as providing a small therapeutic effect on fear avoidance, pain catastrophizing, and functional mobility and sensitivity.[38]

The improvement levels in exercise pain cited above have to be put into the context of the patient's prior pain level and expectations. Imagine a patient who is experiencing a pain level of 8.0 points. At the onset of the management, they are informed that exercise will improve their condition by an average of 1 point, down to a level of approximately 7.0 points. This would be a serious blow for their expectations and a dampener on participation. However, if the individual's starting level is 3.0 points, a drop down to 2.0 points may be more significant.

Perhaps a more important indicator of exercise effectiveness is to ask the patient what they would regard as a meaningful improvement.[39] This can be measured, to a degree, by asking the patient how great the change in pain level would have to be for them to consider it as beneficial and at which level they would consider it to be significantly improved.[40] In chronic low back and neck conditions and frozen shoulder, patients would consider pain improvement above 1.5–2.0 points as relevant.[41-44] Some studies suggest that in low back patients a meaningful change is as high as 3.5–4.7 points in the subacute stage and 2.5–4.5 points in chronic presentations.[45] In the arthritic knee, a meaningful change is between 2.7 and 3.6 points. The symptomatic level at which the patient considers their pain condition to have improved satisfactorily is around 3.0–4.0 points in a wide variety of chronic pain conditions and slightly lower in acute conditions.[40] These cut-off points are stable over time and minimally influenced by age or the condition's duration. These studies imply that the remedial effects of exercise on persistent pain are somewhat low: a lackluster outcome that could partly explain the considerable dropout from lengthy exercise plans.

Overall, exercise has a modest to moderate effect in improving pain and functionality. These overall low-level improvements may seem more appealing if we consider the alternatives: the commonly prescribed pain medications. Exercises are more effective and safer, have no side effects, and carry no danger of addiction. This message is reflected in the recent UK National Institute for Health and Care Excellence (NICE) guidelines, which recommend exercise and physical activities for managing chronic pain and withdrawal from prescribing all forms of ineffective pain medications, including paracetamol, non-steroidal anti-inflammatory drugs, benzodiazepines, or opioids.[46]

The important messages here are: don't leave chronic pain management just to exercise, and don't make pain relief the sole goal of the management. There is more to exercise and being active than the sole outcome of pain alleviation. *Exercise could increase functional engagement, even in the absence of pain alleviation;*

it contributes to physical and cognitive function, sleep, overall health, and quality of life, and helps to reduce disease risk.[47]

> **A sobering thought:** you can only exercise some people out of some pain some of the time – but you are always better off trying.

EXERCISE PRESCRIPTION FOR ACUTE PAIN

The management of acute pain often includes some form of exercise, yet research in this area is very limited.

From an exercise perspective, there are possible top-down or bottom-up processes by which the pain of injury can be alleviated:[48] a top-down modulation, described above, through the effects of exercise on central processes associated with pain; and bottom-up modulation by direct effects of movement on repair processes. As discussed previously (see Chapter 4), mobilization enhances flow through the interstitium and thereby could help regulate the levels of inflammatory cytokines and extent of edema. These may have more immediate and transient effects on the intensity of pain. Additionally, physical activity optimizes the resolution of repair, and may therefore have an overall effect on the duration of pain. It is anticipated that the progression in symptomatic improvements will largely follow the resolution of repair. Hence, physical activities that support repair may indirectly influence the intensity and overall duration of pain.

Generally, all forms of exercise fail to show significant effects in acute pain conditions in terms of pain alleviation or functionality.[37,49–51] Most of these studies have reviewed the role of exercise in acute low back and neck pain. These studies looked specifically at extra-functional exercise, such as stretching, strengthening, aerobics, and so on: a complete mismatch between the underlying condition (potential damage, inflammation) and the physiological attributes of the exercise. More research is needed to explore the role of exercise in managing post-injury and post-surgery pain in various conditions and anatomical locations, perhaps moving away from the strength and conditioning model to more functional management.

MANAGING PAIN: FUNCTIONAL OR EXTRA-FUNCTIONAL?

We are now left with the question: which exercise would be more beneficial – functional or extra-functional?

Pain modulation is a CNS phenomenon. These central processes are likely to be present in both functional and extra-functional activities. Hence, all forms of activities and exercise can be beneficial for managing chronic musculoskeletal pain. This would explain the findings that walking for half an hour daily is as beneficial as specific trunk exercises for managing chronic low back pain.[52] Moreover, the humble walk has been found to be helpful for a range of other persistent pain conditions, including neck pain and osteoarthritis-related knee pain.[32] This means that the individual's own movement repertoire can be utilized to support symptomatic modulation.

There may be additional advantages for a functional approach in managing chronic pain. Let's think for a minute about exercise as a pain medication with a transient analgesic duration. For sustained pain relief, we would expect a person to take the medication several times a day. Similarly, exercise can induce a hypoalgesic effect which could last about 30 minutes (in laboratory conditions); however, exercises are often prescribed and practiced once a day. Perhaps more effective pain control could be achieved by spreading the exercise routine throughout the day.[53] This exposure would be more readily fulfilled by a functional exercise approach. For example, in a pilot study looking at exercise to manage acute pain after knee replacement, it was demonstrated that a 20-minute walk, a day after surgery, provided pain relief that lasted 20 minutes.[48] It would be interesting to see how it would affect pain levels if repeated several times a day. In my clinic, I often recommend frequent short walks several times a day for a wide range of acute and chronic pain conditions. There might be a scheduling advantage for using the more accessible, fuss-free functional activities over extra-functional ones.

Another management consideration is related to the focus of attention and pain. When a person focuses on their pain, they experience it as being more intense, whereas diverting the attention away tends to have an attenuating effect.[54] Extra-functional exercises often contain internal focus-of-attention instructions directed at the body, such as clenching the gluteal muscles, engaging the core, stabilizing the scapula, and so on. A functional exercise approach promotes an external focus which is directed at functional outcomes and away from the body: for example, lift an object off the floor, walk to work, and so on (see Chapter 7). Hence, extra-functional exercise may increase the attention paid to the pain experience, whereas functional activities may help decrease it.

The management itself can become overfocused on the pain experience,[6] particularly if it contains excessive daily schedules and treatment-related tasks, complex postural advice, or a battery of extra-functional exercises that target the painful area. This management would tend to intern the person in an existence that revolves around their pain condition. A solution to overfocus and internal focus can be to minimize the management-related items to the few and the essential, and to shift the exercise prescription away from specific body tissues or a specific body area towards a functional whole-body approach. But is it still effective? Yes: comparable pain reduction has been demonstrated in all forms of exercise, including functional and general exercises, which are likely to be more externally focused.[31,32,55]

> **Clinical application:** in managing chronic low back pain patients, I often apply a "forget the back" approach in which back-specific exercises are replaced with functional activities, such as more walking, carrying shopping, and supporting a return to recreational and sports activities. The focus is external, on the goal of the activity, rather than on correct lifting techniques or engaging specific trunk muscles. It is all about making the person whole using integration rather than fragmentation.

Acute pain: functional or extra-functional?

As discussed elsewhere, the primary role of exercise in acute conditions is to support tissue repair. For this purpose, both functional and extra-functional exercises can be used, as long as they target the affected area (see Chapter 5). There may be some advantage in a functional movement approach, partly because of its simplicity and accessibility to the patient. This was explored in a study that looked at the management of acute low back pain with spinal exercise, bed rest, or maintenance of daily activities within a tolerable level (functional group).[56] After 3 and 12 weeks, the patients in the functional group had better recovery than those prescribed either bed rest or exercises. This was observed in the duration and intensity of pain, range of lumbar flexion, ability to work as measured subjectively, by the Oswestry back-disability index, and number of days absent from work.

Value of the mundane: serendipitously for this chapter, at the time of writing I had two significant injuries. The first was an extremely painful hamstring strain from snagging my foot on a tree root while jogging. It took 3 weeks to be symptom-free and comfortable enough to resume running. In addition to this, "did my back in" lifting a pot in the garden. I experienced severe low back pain complete with antalgic posture and gait. By the end of the first week there was an 80% improvement in symptoms and function, and by the second week the pain was mild enough to reintroduce an attenuated form of jogging (slower and shorter in duration). In both injuries, attenuated walking was used initially to protect and support repair, and gradually amplified in line with the symptomatic improvements. In the two cases, the symptomatic improvements followed the expected duration of repair. I am no hero. The purpose of this report is to highlight that mundane daily functional activities can sometimes be overlooked in exercise prescription; in these examples there was no need for complex back or leg exercises.

SHOULD EXERCISE BE PAINFUL?

The aim of remedial exercise or activity is to bring about a sustained improvement in symptoms, functionality, and quality of life. However, individuals who are already in pain are likely to experience some aggravation of symptoms during and following exercise. This raises the question: at what level and duration is an aggravation of symptoms considered to be beneficial?

In both acute and persistent conditions, pain during exercise may be inevitable. In acute pain conditions, safety considerations guide the intensity of the management. Injuries are likely to be associated with tissue damage and reduced tensile strength, often of unknown magnitude. There is no physiological rationale for high-intensity or painful activities as the means to support repair. High-intensity exercise that inflicts pain may unintentionally result in recurrent damage. In acute conditions the activities should be within a "tolerable discomfort" level and capped with the message "let pain guide you." In chronic pain, exacerbation during and after exercise may be experienced too. The patient should be consulted and monitored to balance the level of activity they can comfortably tolerate in relation to their symptomatic and functional improvement.

Prescribing painful exercise for persistent pain conditions is a complex issue. A recent review of this clinical conundrum suggests that there is a small, though clinically insignificant, advantage for painful over pain-free exercise.[57] The effect is only evident in the short term (up to 3 months). This finding can be viewed in different ways: first, that there is no harm in painful practice, providing that the exercise helps to improve symptoms, functionality, and quality of life. If not, there is no point in pursuing it. Painful management could also help decouple the patient's belief that pain is the consequence of damage.[58] An uncomfortable yet uneventful movement experience can demonstrate to the person that being active is safe. It could reinforce the message that "hurt is not harm." There is support for this approach from behavioral studies of chronic pain and activity repatterning. Chronic pain sufferers who persevere with their often-painful activities benefit most from this attitude in terms of symptoms, functionality, and quality of life.[59,60] Surprisingly, pacing practices for chronic pain, which aim to balance out under- and overdoing behaviors, were shown to have negative effects on pain and functionality, similar to avoidance behavior (see Chapter 13).[59,60] There may be a danger that management that seeks to be pain-free ends up being a race to the functionality bottom, where individuals progressively reduce their activities in the futile search for an existence with least pain. Paradoxically, this negative trajectory is associated with greater pain, depression, future disability, and reduced quality of life. It should be noted that although painful exercises may help alleviate pain,[57] they can dampen adherence to the exercise program.[61]

The success of disassociating pain from injury depends on the patient's capacity to accept and embody this message, which can be very difficult for most people. First, pain plays a protective role in our survival. Pain and behavior are coupled within our non-conscious responses: for example, withdrawing the hand from a hot plate. A person experiencing persistent pain is well aware of this association. Second, throughout life we experience countless injuries, serious illnesses, and medical interventions that result in pain. These lifetime pain-damage experiences strengthen this association, which is not a bad thing for pain of injury. The complication arises in chronic pain, where this association is carried over into what seems to the patient a familiar pain experience: hence the often-observed fear of movement and withdrawal from painful yet safe activities. So, painful exercise can help decouple the pain–harm association but can be a challenging concept for the patient to grasp. Try convincing a person with persistent plantar fasciitis that the painful side is as strong and intact as the non-painful side,

and that walking, running, and jumping may cause more pain but no further damage. For the patient to overcome their fears and beliefs requires an element of courage and an unwavering trust in the therapist.

For some patients, the normalization of painful exercise can be misunderstood and used to justify excessive overuse behavior. This is often linked to the widely held belief that without pain there is no gain, that pain can be extricated by force from the body through intense workouts and use of implements such as rigid foam rollers. When that fails, the frustration with the condition grows, leading to progressively punishing practices towards the body.

Overuse injuries and painful management

Imagine two patients who present with long-term low back pain. One developed the back pain over many months of intensive cycling and the other (non-athlete) developed the condition without an apparent cause. Due to the pain, the cyclist had to withdraw from cycling and the non-athlete had to curtail their walking distance. Two persistent pain conditions – overuse and sensitization. Who would benefit from persevering, regardless of symptoms?

The cyclist may have developed an overuse injury with potential tissue damage. Persevering regardless is contraindicated, as it is likely to worsen the underlying damage, lead to an increase in their symptoms, and further reduce their functionality.[62] Yet, it is very common for athletes to continue training and competing, despite their condition.[63–65] It is not uncommon for the injured athlete to withdraw from their main activity, only to replace it with another demanding activity, such as weight training.[64]

These practices are potentially damaging strategies that are unlikely to help resolve tissue repair. As discussed previously, tissue repair requires a period of activity attenuation, followed by a gradual increase in training intensity.

As for management of the non-athlete, their condition is likely to be associated with persistent sensitization unrelated to tissue damage or repair. They are likely to be safe walking, even if it is uncomfortable or painful. A caveat comes into play here when this management leads to further increases in pain that negatively impact walking and other functional activities.

So often, the remedial management seeks to increase physical engagement in the underactive and moderate it in those who are overactive (as with overuse injuries).[66] However, while implementing activity repatterning sounds simple, it may not be so – it may clash with the patient's habitual pain/illness behavior.[67] The observed pain behavior represents the sum total of past experiences and their interaction with present events. The current pain behavior represents the best solution under the current circumstances. Hence, modifying a person's exercise or functional engagement can be as challenging as changing a person's diet.

MATCHING EXERCISE TO RECOVERY PROCESS

From the individual's perspective, a beneficial pain behavior is the one that provides pain alleviation and enables them to recover their functionality. A person who is in pain is likely to bring to that experience their tried and tested injury/pain behavior, reflected in some form of activity repatterning or specific exercise that worked for them in the past.[68–70] Here, the potential for a mismatch between pain behavior

and actual recovery needs is not unthinkable. It is possible for the individual to engage in movement behavior which is in conflict with the recovery processes: for example, engaging in protective behavior (bed rest) to manage chronic pain which is not associated with tissue damage, or engaging in intense restorative behavior (e.g., stretching) in an acute injury where there is issue damage and loss of tensile strength. In these situations, the individual can be "steered" towards positive movement engagement that supports the underlying recovery process: protective behavior and exercise to support early phases of repair, and restorative behavior to support the latter part of repair and for increasing functional engagement in persistent pain conditions.

EXERCISE AND PAIN ALLEVIATION: IS THERE AN OPTIMAL APPROACH?

An optimal exercise prescription is where training/activity intensity, duration, and frequency produce a lasting improvement in pain relief and functionality. Despite the fact that exercise prescription has been studied extensively over a few decades, we still do not have the answer to this clinical puzzle. There may be several reasons for this. Pain is a highly complex, multidimensional phenomenon and there is no simple exercise solution to fit all possibilities. There are also gaps between research and practice. Optimum methods illuminated by research may not necessarily translate into what is optimum for an individual. By its very nature, research tends to average the data, whereas in clinic the practitioner has to individualize the management with respect to the person's current circumstances. Exercise prescription is a fuzzy-edged, science-informed practice rather than having a precise evidence base.

In past decades, most research has explored exercise prescription through the strength and conditioning lens or a motor control paradigm. This tilt is ubiquitous in current research and systematic reviews.[37,49–51,71,72] It is likely that, by this point, research into these approaches has reached saturation level and any additional studies are unlikely to dramatically change what we already know. In comparison, there is scant research into functional approaches for managing pain conditions. Perhaps it is time to start looking at functional pain management in greater depth.

My educated guess is that optimum pain management can be reached by gradually amplifying the intensity, duration, and frequency of daily activities. We know that we are getting it right when overall pain is diminished and the patient increases their functional engagement.

SUMMARY

- Exercise of any kind can support recovery through symptomatic modulation.

- Using functional activities can be as effective as extra-functional exercise.

- Increasing the intensity, duration, and frequency of exercise can enhance their effects.

- Modulation of pain is associated with biopsychosocial factors rather than structural biomechanical or motor control change.

- In persistent musculoskeletal conditions, both functional and extra-functional exercises have a modest to moderate effect in reducing pain levels, mostly in the short term.

- In acute injuries, being active is essential for optimal healing but may have a limited effect on pain alleviation.

- In persistent conditions, pain is not an indication of tissue damage. Maintaining or increasing the level of activities is safe.

- In acute conditions, pain is an indication of potential damage. Initially, remedial activities should be attenuated and then amplified later using a "let the pain guide you" approach.

- Aggravation of symptoms during exercise may be inevitable in individuals who are already in pain; however, pain should not be applied intentionally as a therapeutic modality.

- There might be advantages to functional over extra-functional exercise for managing pain: the remedial activity is similar to the goals of the management, it can be repeated frequently during the day, and it is readily accessible.

- Since all exercise provides pain alleviation in chronic conditions, use the individual's own movement repertoire. People welcome the idea that they can return to their favorite and much-missed activities.

Chapter 11

References

1. Lazaridou A, Elbaridi N, Edwards RR, Berde CB. Pain assessment. In: Benzon HT, Raja SN, Liu SS, Fishman SM, Cohen SP, editors. Essentials of pain medicine. 4th ed. Edinburgh: Elsevier; 2018.

2. Garland EL. Pain processing in the human nervous system: a selective review of nociceptive and biobehavioral pathways. Prim Care. 2012;39:561–71.

3. Rice D, Nijs J, Kosek E, Widerman T, Hasenbring MI, Koltyn K, et al. Exercise-induced hypoalgesia in pain-free and chronic pain populations: state of the art and future directions. J Pain. 2019;20:1249–66.

4. Nijs J, Kosek E, Van Oosterwijck J, Meeus M. Dysfunctional endogenous analgesia during exercise in patients with chronic pain: to exercise or not to exercise? Pain Physician. 2012;15:ES205–ES213.

5. Fuentes JP, Armijo-Olivo S, Magee DJ, Gross DP. Effects of exercise therapy on endogenous pain-relieving peptides in musculoskeletal pain: a systematic review. Clin J Pain. 2011;27:365–74.

6. Torta DM, Legrain V, Mouraux A, Valentini E. Attention to pain! A neurocognitive perspective on attentional modulation of pain in neuroimaging studies. Cortex. 2017;89:120–34.

7. Legrain V, Perchet C, García-Larrea L. Involuntary orienting of attention to nociceptive events: neural and behavioral signatures. J Neurophysiol. 2009;102:2423–34.

8. Schoth DE, Nunes VD, Liossi C. Attentional bias towards pain-related information in chronic pain; a meta-analysis of visual-probe investigations. Clin Psychol Rev. 2012;32:13–25.

9. Melzack R, Wall PD. Pain mechanisms: a new theory. Science. 1965;150:971–9.

10. Dundar U, Toktas H, Cakir T, Evcik D, Kavuncu V. Continuous passive motion provides good pain control in patients with adhesive capsulitis. Int J Rehab Res. 2009;32:193–8.

11. Willimon SC, Briggs KK, Philippon MJ. Intra-articular adhesions following hip arthroscopy: a risk factor analysis. Knee Surg Sports Traumatol Arthrosc. 2014;22:822–5.

12. Hartvigsen J, Hancock MJ, Kongsted A, Louw Q, Ferreira ML, Genevay S, et al. What low back pain is and why we need to pay attention. Lancet. 2018;391:2356–2367.

13. Hoffman MD, Hoffman DR. Does aerobic exercise improve pain perception and mood? A review of the evidence related to healthy and chronic pain subjects. Curr Pain Headache Rep. 2007;11:93–7.

14. Hurwitz EL, Morgenstern H, Chiao C. Effects of recreational physical activity and back exercises on low back pain and psychological distress: findings from the UCLA Low Back Pain Study. Am J Public Health. 2005;95:1817–24.

15. Ellingson LD, Koltyn KF, Kim JS, Cook DB. Does exercise induce hypoalgesia through conditioned pain modulation? Psychophysiol. 2014;51:267–76.

16. Colloca L, Corsi N, Fiorio M. The interplay of exercise, placebo and nocebo effects on experimental pain. Sci Rep. 2018;8:14758.

17. Koltyn KF. Exercise-induced hypoalgesia and intensity of exercise. Sports Med. 2002;32:477–87.

18. Naugle KM, Naugle KE, Fillingim RB, Samuels B, Riley JL 3rd. Intensity thresholds for aerobic exercise-induced hypoalgesia. Med Sci Sports Exerc. 2014;46:817–25.

19. Naugle KM, Fillingim RB, Riley JL 3rd. A meta-analytic review of the hypoalgesic effects of exercise. J Pain. 2012;13:1139–50.

20. Geva N, Defrin R. Enhanced pain modulation among triathletes: a possible explanation for their exceptional capabilities, Pain. 2013;154:2317–23.

21. Flood A, Waddington G, Thompson K, Cathcart S. Increased conditioned pain modulation in athletes. J Sports Sci. 2017;35:1066–72.

22. Ray CA, Carter JR. Central modulation of exercise-induced muscle pain in humans. J Physiol. 2007;585:287–94.

23. Van Oosterwijck J, Nijs J, Meeus M, van Loo M, Paul L. Lack of endogenous pain inhibition during exercise in people with chronic whiplash associated disorders: an experimental study. J Pain. 2012;13:242–54.

24. Lannersten L, Kosek E. Dysfunction of endogenous pain inhibition during exercise with painful muscles in patients with shoulder myalgia and fibromyalgia. Pain. 2010;151:77–86.

25. Burrows N, Booth J, Sturnieks D, Barry B. Acute resistance exercise and pressure pain sensitivity in knee osteoarthritis: a randomised crossover trial. Osteoarthritis Cartilage. 2014;22:407–14.

26. Qin J, Zhang Y, Wu L, Zexiang H, Huang J, Tao J, et al. Effect of tai chi alone or as additional therapy on low back pain: systematic review and meta-analysis of randomized controlled trials. Medicine (Baltimore). 2019;98:e17099.

27. Kong LJ, Lauche R, Klose P, Bu JH, Yang XC, Guo CQ, et al. Tai chi for chronic pain conditions: a systematic review and meta-analysis of randomized controlled trials. Sci Rep. 2016;6:25325.

28. Landmark T, Romundstad P, Borchgrevink PC, Kaasa S, Dale O. Associations between recreational exercise and chronic pain in the general population: evidence from the HUNT 3 study. Pain. 2011;152:2241–7.

29. Heneweer H, Vanhees L, Picavet SH. Physical activity and low back pain: a U-shaped relation? Pain. 2009;143:21–5.

30. Lear SA, Hu W, Rangarajan S, Gasevic D, Leong D, Iqbal R, et al. The effect of physical activity on mortality and cardiovascular disease in 130 000 people from 17 high-income, middle-income, and low-income countries: the PURE study. Lancet 2017;390:2643–54.

31. Geneen LJ, Moore RA, Clarke C, Martin D, Colvin LA, Smith BH. Physical activity and exercise for chronic pain in adults: an overview of Cochrane Reviews.

Cochrane Database Syst Rev. 2017;4:CD011279.

32. O'Connor SR, Tully MA, Ryan B, Bleakley CM, Baxter GD, Bradley JM, et al. Walking exercise for chronic musculoskeletal pain: systematic review and meta-analysis. Arch Phys Med Rehab. 2015;96:724–34.

33. Owen PJ, Miller CT, Mundell NL, Verswijveren SJ, Tagliaferri SD, Brisby H, et al. Which specific modes of exercise training are most effective for treating low back pain? Network meta-analysis. Br J Sports Med. 2020;54:1279–87.

34. Wylde V, Dennis J, Gooberman-Hill R, Beswick AD. Effectiveness of postdischarge interventions for reducing the severity of chronic pain after total knee replacement: systematic review of randomised controlled trials. BMJ Open. 2018;8:e020368.

35. Fransen M, McConnell S, Harmer AR, Van der Esch M, Simic M, Bennell KL. Exercise for osteoarthritis of the knee. Cochrane Database Syst Rev. 2015 Jan 9;1:CD004376.

36. Fransen M, McConnell S, Hernandez-Molina G, Reichenbach S. Exercise for osteoarthritis of the hip. Cochrane Database Syst Rev. 2014 Apr 22;4:CD007912.

37. Hayden JA, van Tulder MW, Malmivaara A, Koes BW. Exercise therapy for treatment of non-specific low back pain. Cochrane Database Syst Rev 2005;3:CD000335.

38. Louw A, Goldrick S, Bernstetter A, Van Gelder LH, Parr A, Zimney K, et al. Evaluation is treatment for low back pain, J Man Manip

Ther. 2021;29:4–13. Epub 2020 Feb 24.

39. Tubach F, Dougados M, Falissard B, Baron G, Logeart I, Ravaud P. Feeling good rather than feeling better matters more to patients. Arthritis Rheum. 2006;55:526–30.

40. Kvien TK, Heiberg T, Hagen KB. Minimal clinically important improvement/difference (MCII/MCID) and patient acceptable symptom state (PASS): what do these concepts mean? Ann Rheum Dis. 2007;66 Suppl 3:iii40–iii41.

41. Kovacs FM, Abraira V, Royuela A, Corcoll J, Alegre L, Cano A, et al. Minimal clinically important change for pain intensity and disability in patients with nonspecific low back pain. Spine (Phila Pa 1976). 2007;32:2915–20.

42. Kovacs FM, Abraira V, Royuela A, Corcoll J, Alegre L, Tomás M, et al. Minimum detectable and minimal clinically important changes for pain in patients with nonspecific neck pain. BMC Musculoskelet Disord. 2008;9:43.

43. Tashjian RZ. Minimal clinically important differences (MCID) and patient acceptable symptomatic state (PASS) for visual analog scales (VAS) measuring pain in patients treated for rotator cuff disease. J Shoulder Elbow Surg. 2009;18:927–32.

44. Hawker GA, Mian S, Kendzerska T, French M. Measures of adult pain: Visual Analog Scale for Pain (VAS Pain), Numeric Rating Scale for Pain (NRS Pain), McGill Pain Questionnaire (MPQ), Short-Form McGill Pain

Questionnaire (SF-MPQ), Chronic Pain Grade Scale (CPGS), Short Form-36 Bodily Pain Scale (SF-36 BPS), and Measure of Intermittent and Constant Osteoarthritis Pain (ICOAP). Arthritis Care Res. 2011;63:S240–S252.

45. van der Roer N, Ostelo RWJG, Bekkering GE, van Tulder MW, de Vet HCW. Minimal clinically important change for pain intensity, functional status, and general health status in patients with nonspecific low back pain. Spine. 2006;31:578–82.

46. NICE guideline [NG193]. Chronic pain (primary and secondary) in over 16s: assessment of all chronic pain and management of chronic primary pain; National Institute for Health and Care Excellence; 2021. Available from: https://www.nice.org.uk/guidance/ng193/chapter/Recommendations.

47. Ambrose KR, Golightly YM. Physical exercise as non-pharmacological treatment of chronic pain: why and when. Best Pract Res Clin Rheumatol. 2015;29:120–30.

48. Lunn TH, Kristensen BB, Gaarn-Larsen L, Kehlet H. Possible effects of mobilisation on acute post-operative pain and nociceptive function after total knee arthroplasty. Acta Anaesthesiol Scand. 2012;56:1234–40.

49. Gross A, Kay TM, Paquin JP, Blanchette S, Lalonde P, Christie T, et al. Exercises for mechanical neck disorders. Cochrane Database Syst Rev. 2015 Jan 28;1:CD004250.

50. Macedo LG, Saragiotto BT, Yamato TP, Costa LOP, Menezes Costa LC, Ostelo RWJG, et al. Motor control exercise for acute non-specific low back pain. Cochrane Database Syst Rev. 2016;2:CD012085.

51. Faas A, Chavannes AW, van Eijk JT, Gubbels JW. A randomized, placebo-controlled trial of exercise therapy in patients with acute low back pain. Spine. 1993;18:1388–95.

52. van Middelkoop M, Rubinstein SM, Verhagen AP, Ostelo RW, Koes BW, van Tulder MW. Exercise therapy for chronic nonspecific low-back pain. Best Pract Res Clin Rheumatol. 2010;24:193–204.

53. Polaski AM, Phelps AL, Kostek MC, Szucs KA, Kolber BJ. Exercise-induced hypoalgesia: a meta-analysis of exercise dosing for the treatment of chronic pain. PLoS One. 2019;14:e0210418.

54. Sprenger C, Eippert F, Finsterbusch J, Bingel U, Rose M, Büchel C. Attention modulates spinal cord responses to pain. Curr Biol. 2012;22:1019–22.

55. de Zoete RMJ, Brown L, Oliveira K, Penglaze L, Rex R, Sawtell B, et al. The effectiveness of general physical exercise for individuals with chronic neck pain: a systematic review of randomised controlled trials. Eur J Physiother. 2020;22141–7.

56. Malmivaara A, Häkkinen U, Aro T, Heinrichs ML, Koskenniemi L, Kuosma E, et al. The treatment of acute low back pain: bed rest, exercises, or ordinary activity? N Engl J Med. 1995;332:351–5.

57. Smith BE, Hendrick P, Smith TO, Bateman M, Moffatt F, Rathleff MS, et al. Should exercises be painful in the management of chronic musculoskeletal pain? A systematic review and meta-analysis. Br J Sports Med. 2017;51:1679–87.

58. Smith BE, Hendrick P, Bateman M, Holden S, Littlewood C, Smith TO, et al. Musculoskeletal pain and exercise—challenging existing paradigms and introducing new. Br J Sports Med. 2019;53:907–12.

59. Kindermans HP, Roelofs J, Goossens ME, Huijnen IP, Verbunt JA, Vlaeyen JW. Activity patterns in chronic pain: underlying dimensions and associations with disability and depressed mood. J Pain. 2011;12:1049–58.

60. Andrews NE, Strong J, Meredith PJ, Gordon K, Bagraith KS. "It's very hard to change yourself": an exploration of overactivity in people with chronic pain using interpretative phenomenological analysis. Pain. 2015;156:1215–31.

61. Jack K, McLean SM, Moffett JK, Gardiner E. Barriers to treatment adherence in physiotherapy outpatient clinics: a systematic review. Man Ther. 2010;15:220–8.

62. Clarsen B, Krosshaug T, Bahr R. Overuse injuries in professional road cyclists. Am J Sports Med. 2010;38:2494–501.

63. Harringe ML, Lindblad S, Werner S. Do team gymnasts compete in spite of symptoms from an injury? Br J Sports Med. 2004;38:398–401.

64. Vleck VE, Bentley DJ, Millet GP, Cochrane T. Triathlon event distance specialization: training and injury effects. J Strength Cond Res. 2010;24:30–6.

65. Myklebust G, Hasslan L, Bahr R, Steffen K. High prevalence of shoulder pain among elite Norwegian female handball players. Scand J Med Sci Sports. 2013;233:288–94.

66. Luthi F, Vuistiner P, Favre C, Hilfiker R, Léger B. Avoidance, pacing, or persistence in multidisciplinary functional rehabilitation for chronic musculoskeletal pain: an observational study with cross-sectional and longitudinal analyses. PLoS One. 2018;13:e0203329.

67. Andrews NE, Strong J, Meredith PJ. Overactivity in chronic pain: is it a valid construct? Pain. 2015;156:1991–2000.

68. Keefe F, Pryor R. Assessment of pain behaviors. In: Schmidt R, Willis W, editors. Encyclopedia of pain. Berlin and Heidelberg; Springer; 2007.

69. Murphy SL, Kratz AL. Activity pacing in daily life: a within-day analysis. Pain. 2014;155:2630–7.

70. Antcliff D, Keenan AM, Keeley P, Woby S, McGowan L. Survey of activity pacing across healthcare professionals informs a new activity pacing framework for chronic pain/ fatigue. Musculoskeletal Care. 2019;17:335–45.

71. Price J, Rushton A, Tyros I, Tyros V, Heneghan NR. Effectiveness and optimal dosage of exercise training for chronic non-specific neck pain: a systematic review with a narrative synthesis. PLoS One. 2020;15:e0234511.

72. Robinson A, McIntosh J, Peberdy H, Wishart D, Brown G, Pope H, et al. The effectiveness of physiotherapy interventions on pain and quality of life in adults with persistent post-surgical pain compared to usual care: a systematic review. PLoS One. 2019;14:e0226227.

Chapter 12

Contents
Exercise prescription for management of stiffness

A patient complains about localized stiffness due to an ankle sprain, a different patient has severe stiffness and range of movement (ROM) losses after lower limb immobilizations, and another is a chronic low back pain sufferer complaining of severe localized spinal stiffness in the morning.

Stiffness is a common symptom observed in musculoskeletal practice; often, where there is pain there is likely to be some form of stiffness, but frequently stiffness may be the only presenting symptom. Not all stiffness is the same and hence exercise prescription has to take into account the underlying causes and physiological processes that give rise to this symptom.

Before delving into the management of stiffness with exercise, though, we need to consider what stiffness is and how it relates to ROM.

STIFFNESS AND RANGE OF MOVEMENT

Range of movement and stiffness are two different things. ROM is how far a joint can be moved, either actively or passively. Stiffness, confusingly, is related to two different and somewhat connected phenomena. There is biomechanical stiffness, which is the resistance measured when a tissue is put under a stretching force;[1] for example, a ligament is stiffer than a muscle. This biomechanical property can be measured on a tissue sample in a laboratory. When tested on a conscious subject, however, a felt experience of stiffness is introduced – the growing resistance discomfort felt when we bring a joint to its end-range. This sensation arises from excitation of local mechanoreceptors and the transmission and processing of these signals centrally, culminating in the experience of stiffness. Overall, the

role of felt stiffness is protective, alerting us to impending damage.[2]

Biomechanical stiffness can be demonstrated by passively extending your index finger to the end-range; hold that angle for a few moments, release it and then restretch it to the end-range. If the experiment was successful, there would be an increase in the range while less stiffness was experienced (Fig. 12.1A). This is partly due to the viscoelastic properties of tissues, which become more compliant (less stiff) under repeated loading.[3] This change in tissue stiffness is transient and tends to revert to the pre-stretching level. In the hamstrings it recovers within an hour, while in the Achilles tendon it will take several hours.[4,5]

However, there is a twist in the stiffness tale. It has been demonstrated that an acute bout of hamstring stretching on one side increases the range on the other unstretched side.[6] Similarly, an acute bout of shoulder joint stretching increases the ROM in the unstretched hip and vice versa.[7] The range increase in the unstretched joints cannot be explained as tissue change or modification in the local receptors or transmission of the signals centrally. Therefore, we have to assume that it is a central process – probably a psychological–contextual response. In the absence of injury, there is no threat and therefore stretching is conceived of as being safe. Hence, the person becomes overall *stretch-tolerant*, regardless of the anatomical location of the stretching (Fig. 12.1B). We can also assume that the person may become *stretch-averse* if the end-range is associated with harm, whether real or anticipated.[2] So, a person's experience of stiffness and ROM can be influenced by psychological factors, and not just by biomechanics.

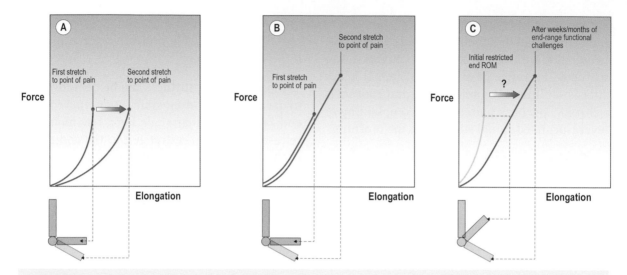

FIGURE 12.1

Possible mechanisms in range of movement (ROM) improvements. (A) Transient biomechanical change in ROM due to viscoelastic change in stiffness – same force resulting in greater elongation, depicted as a right shift in the stiffness curve (orange arrow). (B) A stretch tolerance model in which stiffness remains unchanged (no right shift) but the person becomes more tolerant to discomfort or pain during stretching. (C) Recovery of ROM by tissue adaptation, such as following immobilization. This could be related to a biomechanical restoration of tissue length and extensibility, with or without a change in stiffness (right shift). It is likely that stretch tolerance, stretch desensitization, and adaptation play a role in long-term recovery from tissue-related ROM losses. (For further discussion see Lederman E. Therapeutic stretching: towards a functional approach. Edinburgh: Churchill Livingstone; 2013[13]).

STIFFNESS AS A SYMPTOM

There are several causes behind the experience of stiffness. In essence, this symptom can arise from peripheral, tissue-related causes or as a central nervous system (CNS) phenomenon. The main peripheral causes are inflammation and swelling, often seen following acute injuries, surgery, and lymphedema. Another is the stiffness experienced due to loss of tissue extensibility, such as that seen following immobilization. There are also long-term CNS contributions to the experience of stiffness that are not related to tissue damage or change in biomechanical properties.

Injury, stiffness, and stretch sensitivity

Stiffness is a common experience in injury and, like pain, has a positive protective role. Following injury, there is a drop in the tensile strength of the damaged tissue with a corresponding increase in the experience of stiffness – the perception of an increase in tension sensation in ranges that were previously asymptomatic and out of awareness. This "stretchy pain" experience is referred to as *stretch sensitivity*. The exaggerated felt stiffness is essentially a warning signal that the tissues are being loaded in an unfavorable way. The source of this sensation is probably the distention of local tissues by edema, combined with sensitization of local nociceptors by inflammation, and a possible contribution from central sensitization (see Chapter 10). The outcome is an increase in mechanosensitivity of the local receptors, reflected in the experience of stretch sensitivity. This sensitivity is likely to peak around the inflammatory phase and will gradually diminish as the repair process progresses.

Delayed-onset muscle soreness (DOMS) after exercise is another common cause of stiffness and ROM losses. The experienced stiffness is due to a combination of tissue-related processes and central mechanisms, including an increase in the fluid content of the muscle (a 5% increase in muscle volume increases mechanical stiffness by 10%), damage-related contractures in the muscle fiber, and neural sensitization (stretch sensitivity).[8–10] The felt stiffness tends to diminish over a few days in line with recovery from DOMS.

Biomechanical stiffness

Adaptive changes in tissue morphology and material properties can give rise to biomechanical stiffness and ROM losses.[1] Reduced tissue extensibility is commonly observed following immobilization, in post-surgical adhesions, and in advanced age. The tissue changes associated with biomechanical stiffness have been discussed extensively in Chapter 4. Other disorders can give rise to biomechanical stiffness, such as autoimmune conditions (for example, scleroderma) Dupuytren's contracture,[11] frozen shoulder,[12] CNS damage, and more. However, and importantly, loss of extensibility does not occur spontaneously in the body – people do not lose their biomechanical extensibility overnight. For such adaptive changes to occur, a person would have to be immobilized for a few weeks or suffer from a condition that would in time stiffen them up. Contrary to popular belief, reduced extensibility does not arise from a lack of physical activity, absence of stretching exercise, or poor posture.[13] For example, there is a widely held belief that sitting hunched over a computer will shorten the pectoral muscles. Luckily, that does not happen;[14] otherwise, the posture of office workers would be permanently formed into the shape of their chairs.

Stretch sensitivity and stiffness

Let's go back for a minute to the pain of sensitization (see Chapter 10), the phenomenon where pain can persist long after tissue healing has taken place and is sustained by CNS processes. It could be that, through similar processes, stretch sensitivity can persist long after an injury.

Persistent stretch sensitivity is fascinating and counter-intuitive. Individuals with chronic back pain often complain of raised stiffness in the back of their thighs when bending forward. When examined and compared to pain-free individuals, they exhibit reduced hamstring extensibility (biomechanical elongation) and hip flexion ROM during a straight-leg test. However, there is no difference in biomechanical stiffness of the hamstrings between the groups.[15] Hence, the ROM and extensibility losses were determined by the individual's stretch tolerance, a central process, rather than by biomechanical stiffness. This phenomenon can be observed in the spine. Chronic back pain sufferers often report being stiff in their back but it is unclear if this is due to perceived or "real" biomechanical stiffness (feeling stiff versus being stiff).

Using a specialized spinal stiffness measuring device, it was demonstrated that back pain sufferers and pain-free individuals have the same biomechanical spinal stiffness, although back sufferers reported feeling stiffer than their pain-free controls.[2] Interestingly, amputees are known to experience phantom pain but they can also experience phantom joint stiffness in the missing limb.[16] The symptoms of phantom stiffness respond to imaginary exercise of the phantom limb. So, the brain and memory have a great part to play in the sensation of stiffness.

These studies demonstrate the difference between feeling stiff and being stiff, and that this experience is heightened and sustained in the presence of persistent pain conditions. Similar to the pain of sensitivity, stretch sensitivity is a biopsychosocial and behavioral phenomenon. The tightness in the back of the thighs experienced by a person with acute back pain when they bend forward is a useful warning signal that flexion overloading of damaged spinal tissues is taking place. However, a person with chronic back pain may feel a similar tightness when bending forward, although there is no underlying damage. This may be a reflection of the struggle of the CNS/individual to differentiate between the pain-stiffness of injury and the pain-stiffness of sensitization.

It is possible for stretch sensitivity to be present with biomechanical stiffness. For example, after removal of a plaster cast there is biomechanical stiffness due to loss of extensibility, often combined with pain and heightened stretch sensitivity.

EXERCISE FOR STIFFNESS

Apart from stretching, there is very little research into the management of stiffness with exercise. An important consideration in exercise management is that stiffness is a symptom.

To alleviate it, we need to identify and manage its cause. This brings us back to the three case presentations from the beginning of the chapter. In the patient complaining of localized stiffness due to a recent ankle sprain: this presentation is associated with injury-related stiffness due to swelling and sensitization. The person with severe stiffness and ROM losses after immobilizations is experiencing loss of tissue extensibility, potential complications from adhesion, and local sensitization (Fig. 12.1C). The chronic low back pain sufferer is likely to experience stiffness-associated stretch sensitivity, which is a central process. Each of these presentations will need specific exercise management.

Exercise and injury stiffness

In injury, stretch sensitivity heightens the experience of stiffness or tightness, leading to a perception that the damaged tissues have shortened. Often, individuals take up vigorous stretching exercise to elongate these perceived restrictions. However, and importantly, in acute injuries the affected tissues are likely to have been pulled apart and damaged. They do not somehow undergo biomechanical shortening, unless immobilized. This means that, in acute injuries, stretching exercises, which aim to elongate tissue, will be unhelpful and are potentially damaging: nothing is shortened and there is nothing to stretch. From an exercise perspective, the advice could be: don't stretch your acute injuries. Instead, "pump" the affected tissues with repetitive, cyclical functional/extra-functional activities (see Chapter 5).[17] This can be achieved by simply maintaining the shared activities within tolerable ranges and gradually amplifying them in line with improvements (see Chapter 9).

Generally, exercise management of injury-related stiffness is not well researched. More work is needed, particularly in post-surgical care of edema, where excessive swelling can impede the rate of recovery and endanger the surgical repair.

Exercise to improve extensibility and ROM

Stretching exercises are universally and almost exclusively recommended for reducing stiffness and recovering extensibility and ROM. However, extensive research has demonstrated that several weeks of stretching fail to deliver any significant improvement in ROM. The effect on joint mobility was a mere increase of 3° immediately after stretching, 1° in the short term, and 0° in the long term.[18] This outcome was found across all stretching methods and a wide range of conditions associated with ROM loss. However, we do not know what happens after many months of stretching. How do dancers and yoga practitioners achieve their remarkable flexibility?

The consequence of this research on stretching is that we do not know what can help in clinic – is it possible to expedite functional ROM recovery? To resolve this, we need to consider how daily ROM is maintained in individuals who do not stretch. We can speculate that the forces generated by daily activities load our

tissue to levels that maintain the functional ranges; hence, functional loading supports functional ROM (Fig. 12.2). Then comes the observation that, over time, people do recover from post-immobilization ROM losses simply by being active. But would these activities generate enough loading forces required for tissue adaptation? For example, would walking and using the stairs help restore dorsiflexion ROM following ankle immobilization? The forces generated through the ankle and foot can be surprisingly high in walking. Ground reaction force in the ankle and foot during walking is 2.5–4 × body weight (BW) and the calf muscles exert a force of approximately 2.5×BW.[19] These are likely to be much higher during fast walking and use of stairs. Furthermore, the loss of extensibility in immobilization and its recovery during remobilization is related to adaptive processes (see Chapter 7). The training conditions that drive adaptation are specificity (walk), overloading (walk faster, use stairs), and repetition (walk more). Hence, a manageable daily walk of 3,000–6,000 steps could provide 1500–3000 high-load, stretch-like repetitions on the affected tissues. It could explain how individuals who are physically active recover from their (ankle) ROM losses.[20]

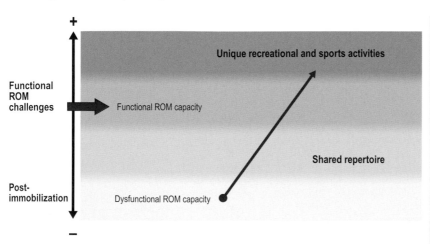

FIGURE 12.2
Functional ROM challenges maintain functional ROM capacity. Functional ROM recovery may be achieved by increasing the end-range movement challenges during the day.

This recovery is associated with normalization of biomechanical stiffness that may take several months.[21] Overall ROM improvement following immobilization could be the combination of being and feeling less stiff.

ROM rehabilitation by amplifying end-range movement during daily activities is discussed in Chapter 8 (see component-focused rehabilitation). A full exploration of this approach can be found in my book *Therapeutic Stretching: Towards a Functional Approach.*[13]

Exercise for stretch sensitivity/chronic stiffness

The fact that individuals can experience stiffness without underlying loss of biomechanical extensibility has important implications for exercise prescription. Most patients will associate this symptom with tissue tightening and, accordingly, attempt to stretch the affected area. However, it is unlikely that stretching exercise will help to alleviate this symptom because there is nothing to loosen up or re-elongate. Furthermore, it is well established that all forms of stretching have no clinically significant effect on pain.[22,23] Assuming that persistent pain and stiffness share similar perceptual–psychological processes, we can speculate that stretching exercises are unlikely to have an effect on stretch sensitivity.

Unfortunately, due to the scant research in this area we do not know which exercise or activities can alleviate persistent stiffness or stretch sensitivity. From my own clinical observations and patients' reports, stiffness seems to be relieved by movement – any movement. Often, patients will report that low back stiffness in the morning or after prolonged sitting dissipates once they are up and moving around. Being active seems to be safe and beneficial for individuals experiencing persistent stretch sensitivity.

Table 12.1 summarizes the different causes of stiffness experiences and their management with exercise.

Table 12.1 Causes of stiffness experience and their management with exercise				
Condition	Swelling	Stretch sensitivity	Reduced tissue extensibility	Exercise management
Injury	✓	✓		Activities consisting of repetitive and cyclical movement
Sensitization		✓		Functional and extra-functional (within tolerable discomfort)
Delayed-onset muscle soreness (DOMS)	✓	✓		
Immobilization		✓	✓	End-range functional activities (may be painful but safe)
Advanced age			✓	
Autoimmune conditions (scleroderma)			✓	?
Other (e.g., Dupuytren's contracture)			✓	

SUMMARY

- Stiffness is a common symptom observed in musculoskeletal conditions.

- Stiffness can be biomechanical (being stiff) and perceptual–psychological phenomenon (feeling stiff).

- Stretch sensitivity is a raised experience of stiffness, disproportionate to mechanical stiffness.

- Stretch sensitivity is likely to be present in all stiffness-related conditions, acute or chronic.

- Biomechanical stiffness may be absent in chronic pain conditions.

- Stiffness associated with injury and chronic pain conditions could be managed with movement – functional or extra-functional.

- Biomechanical stiffness, such as post-immobilization, may be assisted by functional stretching – amplifying end-ranges during daily activities.

- Stretching is not effective in alleviating or treating the causes of stiffness.

- More research is needed to explore the management of stiffness with activity and exercise (anyone for a PhD?).

References

1. Trudel G, Uhthoff HK, Brown M. Extent and direction of joint motion limitation after prolonged immobility: an experimental study in the rat. Arch Phys Med Rehabil. 1999;80:1542–7.

2. Stanton TR, Moseley GL, Wong AYL, Kawchuk GN. Feeling stiffness in the back: a protective perceptual inference in chronic back pain. Sci Rep. 2017;7:9681.

3. Magnusson SP. Passive properties of human skeletal muscle during stretch maneuvers. A review. Scand J Med Sci Sports. 1998;8:65–77.

4. Magnusson SP, Simonsen EB, Dyhre-Poulsen P, Aagaard P, Mohr T, Kjaer M. Viscoelastic stress relaxation during static stretch in human skeletal muscle in the absence of EMG activity. Scand J Med Sci Sports. 1996;6:323–8.

5. Duong B, Low M, Moseley AM, Lee RYW, Herbert RD. Time course of stress relaxation and recovery in human ankles. Clin Biomech. 2001;16:601–7.

6. Chaouachi A, Padulo J, Kasmi S, Othmen AB, Chatra M, Behm DG. Unilateral static and dynamic hamstrings stretching increases contralateral hip flexion range of motion. Clin Physiol Funct Imaging. 2017;37:23–9.

7. Behm DG, Cavanaugh T, Quigley P, Reid JC, Nardi PS, Marchetti PH., Acute bouts of upper and lower body static and dynamic stretching increase non-local joint range of motion. Eur J Appl Physiol. 2016;116:241–9.

8. Sleboda DA, Wold ES, Roberts TJ. Passive muscle tension increases in proportion to intramuscular fluid volume. J Exp Biol. 2019;222:jeb209668.

9. Whitehead NP, Weerakkody NS, Gregory JE, Morgan DL, Proske U. Changes in passive tension of muscle in humans and animals after eccentric exercise. J Physiol. 2001;533:593–604.

10. Proske U. Muscle tenderness from exercise: mechanisms? J Physiol. 2005;564:1.

11. Ball C, Izadi D, Verjee LS, Chan J, Nanchahal J. Systematic review of non-surgical treatments for early Dupuytren's disease. BMC Musculoskelet Disord. 2016;17:345.

12. Kanazawa K, Hagiwara Y, Sekiguchi T, Suzuki K, Koide M, Ando A, et al. Correlations between capsular changes and ROM restriction in frozen shoulder evaluated by plain MRI and MR arthrography. Open Orthop J. 2018; 12:396–404.

13. Lederman E. Therapeutic stretching: towards a functional approach. Edinburgh: Churchill Livingstone; 2013.

14. Hrysomallis C, Goodman C. A review of resistance exercise and posture realignment. J Strength Cond Res. 2001;15:385–90.

15. Halbertsma JP, Göeken LN, Hof AL, Groothoff JW, Eisma WH. Extensibility and stiffness of the hamstrings in patients with nonspecific low back pain. Arch Phys Med Rehabil. 2001;82:232–8.

16. Haigh RC, McCabe CS, Halligan PW, Blake DR. Joint stiffness in a phantom limb: evidence of central nervous system involvement in rheumatoid arthritis. Rheumatol. 2003;42: 888–92.

17. Crawford ME. Surgical complications and their treatments. In: Dock Dockery G, Crawford ME. Lower extremity soft tissue and cutaneous plastic surgery. 2nd ed. Edinburgh: Elsevier; 2012. pp. 435–45.

18. Katalinic OM, Harvey LA, Herbert RD, Moseley AM, Lannin NA, Schurr K. Stretch for the treatment and prevention of contractures. Cochrane Database Syst Rev. 2010 Sep 8;9:CD007455.

19. Rodgers MM. Dynamic biomechanics of the normal foot and ankle during walking and running. Phys Ther. 1988;68:1822–30.

20. Moseley AM, Herbert RD, Nightingale EJ, Taylor DA, Evans TM, Robertson GJ, et al. Passive stretching does not enhance outcomes in patients with plantarflexion contracture after cast immobilization for ankle fracture: a randomized controlled trial. Arch Phys Med Rehabil. 2005;86:1118–26.

21. Nightingale EJ, Moseley AM, Herbert RD. Passive dorsiflexion flexibility after cast immobilization for ankle fracture. Clin Orthop Relat Res. 2007;456:65–9.

22. Harvey LA, Katalinic OM, Herbert RD, Moseley AM, Lannin NA, Schurr K. Stretch for the treatment and prevention of contractures. Cochrane Database Syst Rev. 2017 Jan 9;1:CD007455.

23. Herbert RD, de Noronha M, Kamper SJ. Stretching to prevent or reduce muscle soreness after exercise. Cochrane Database Syst Rev. 2011 Jul 6;7:CD004577.

In this part of the book you will explore:

- The shared management
- How it can be applied to enhance participation in remedial activities

Part 5
Putting it all together

Chapter 13

ADHERENCE

Imagine that you are prescribing a set of remedial exercises or activities that are essential for functional recovery. What would promote adherence and what would limit it? There are numerous factors which can affect exercise/activity adherence (Table 13.1). The constellation of these factors can be likened to a dynamic jigsaw puzzle with adherence attributes spanning multiple dimensions, including biological, psychological, social and cultural, environmental, and the characteristics of the prescribed physical activities.

Table 13.1 Summary of the factors associated with overall physical activity in adults.

Type	Examples	Association
Demographic and biological factors	Age	– –
	Blue-collar occupation	+
	Childlessness	+
	Education	+ +
	Gender (male)	+ +
	Hereditary factors	+ +
	High risk for heart disease	–
	Income/socioeconomic status	+
	Injury history	+
	Marital status (married)	0
	Overweight/obesity	– –
	Race/ethnicity (non-white)	–
Physical, cognitive, and emotional factors	Attitudes	00
	Barriers to exercise	– –
	Control over exercise	+
	Enjoyment of exercise	+ +
	Expectation of benefits	+ +
	Health locus of control	0
	Intention to exercise	+ +
	Knowledge of health and exercise	00
	Lack of time	– –
	Mood disturbance	– –
	Normative beliefs	00
	Perceived health or fitness	+ +
	Personality variables	+
	Poor body image	–
	Psychological health	+
	Self-efficacy	+ +
	Self-motivation	+ +
	Self-schemata for exercise	+ +
	Stage of change	+ +
	Stress	0
	Susceptibility to illness/seriousness of illness	00
	Value of exercise outcomes	0

Table 13.1 (Continued)

Type	Examples	Association
Behavioral attributes and skills	Activity history during childhood/youth	0
	Activity history during adulthood	+ +
	Alcohol	0
	Contemporary exercise program	0
	Dietary habits (quality)	+ +
	Past exercise program	+ +
	Processes of change	+ +
	School sports	0
	Skills for coping with barriers	+
	Smoking	–
	Sports media use	0
	Type A behavior pattern	+
	Decisional balance sheet	+
Social and cultural factors	Class size	ND
	Exercise models	0
	Group cohesion	ND
	Past family influences	0
	Physician influence	+ +
	Social isolation	–
	Social support from friends/peers	+ +
	Social support from spouse/family	+ +
	Social support from staff/instructor	ND
Physical environment factors	Access to facilities: actual	+
	Access to facilities: perceived	+
	Adequate lighting	0
	Climate/season	– –
	Cost of programs	0
	Disruptions in routine	ND
	Enjoyable scenery	+
	Frequent observation of others exercising	+
	Heavy traffic	0
	Home equipment	+
	High crime rates in region	0
	Hilly terrain	+
	Neighborhood safety	+
	Presence of sidewalks	0
	Satisfaction with facilities	+
	Unattended dogs	0
	Urban location	–

Continued

Here are some considerations that could assist adherence within the functional dimension:

- *Use patient-centered goals:* focus on goals that are important to the patient (being able to bend and slip on their sock) and less on clinical goals (have a strong core).[12,24,25] To identify patients' management goals, they can be asked: "What would you consider a successful outcome of the exercise/ rehabilitation/treatment/management?"

- *Empower self-efficacy and autonomy:* keep the patient (positively) informed about their condition and about how their participation can help the recovery processes,[12,26–30] for example, by saying that being active helps tissue healing and strength. Empowerment can be further supported by consulting and involving the patient in developing the movement challenge, including the activities targeted, the scheduling of exposure, and the setting of short- and long-term goals and time scales for the return to activity.[31]

- *Give challenges, not exercise:* I tend to use the phrase "daily challenges" rather than exercise, particularly with individuals who are exercise-shy. Additionally, the term "exercise" may be negatively associated with previous experiences where the person has failed to maintain exercise routines.

- *Make the challenges readily accessible:*[24,32] the notion of exercise is often associated with activities that require set-aside time, use of specialized equipment, and a dedicated location, such as a gym.[33] In a functional approach, the challenges are part of the patient's daily repertoire. They are incorporated into the individual's home, work, and recreational activities. This approach brings

the care within reach of the individual's environment.[10,24]

- *Keep it simple:* avoid complex management protocols or exercises. Simple routines tend to increase compliance.[34] Individuals often find it difficult to recall instructions and advice.[35] Hence, it is helpful to keep the advice and plan concise and simple, and to recap in subsequent sessions.[12] Patients who understand the management concepts are more able to translate the advice to modify and develop their own personalized exercise and lifestyle changes that sustain the remedial program.[11]

- *Provide ongoing support and feedback:*[12,22] recovery can be a very lonely journey without companionship. Ongoing support and feedback can increase adherence behavior.

- *Make it fun:* the element of enjoyment is also important for exercise adherence. It is useful to create a wish-list of activities that the individual enjoys and would like to return to. These sports/physical activities are the remedial exercises.[11]

AVOIDANCE BEHAVIOR

When we are injured or in pain, there is a natural fear that movement may increase the pain intensity or cause further damage.[36] In response, we may avoid certain ranges of movement or withdraw from activities which we believe to be aggravating or harmful.[37–45] The outcome is lower engagement in activities which otherwise would be beneficial for our functional recovery and well-being.

Activity avoidance can be seen as a useful natural protection strategy when viewed from an injury perspective. However, avoidance can be disproportional to the actual level of damage, particularly in chronic musculoskeletal pain conditions (see Chapter 10). For example, in patients with acute and chronic low back pain, pain-related fears and catastrophizing can be more indicative of their physical ability to lift than pain intensity itself.[46,47] Fear of re-injury has been found to play a major role in delaying a return to sports after anterior cruciate ligament reconstruction. An increased fear of movement was associated with worse knee pain and quality of life 2–4 years after surgery.[48] Hence, the fear of pain and re-injury can be more disabling than the pain or the condition itself. [44,49]

There are several factors that can feed avoidance behavior.[50] It can arise from exposure to inaccurate, misleading, or conflicting information about the condition and how to manage it – a cognitive form of avoidance (misinformed avoiders). Activity avoidance

can also come about through a learned association between pain and movement (learned pain avoiders), which could outlast recovery and may affect activities which are not related to the original injury.[42,50] For example, patients who recover from back pain may maintain restricted, antalgic-like movement strategies, even when they have mild symptoms or are pain-free.[42]

Fear avoidance can also come about when a person transfers their fears and anxieties from another aspect of their life to their current musculoskeletal or pain condition (affective avoiders).[50] This can happen in individuals who suffer from general anxiety or depressive states.[51,52] This phenomenon was demonstrated in a large population study on whiplash injury. Individuals who exhibit more fear avoidance, who were anxious and depressed, or who displayed negative illness behavior *pre-injury* were more likely to report whiplash injury,

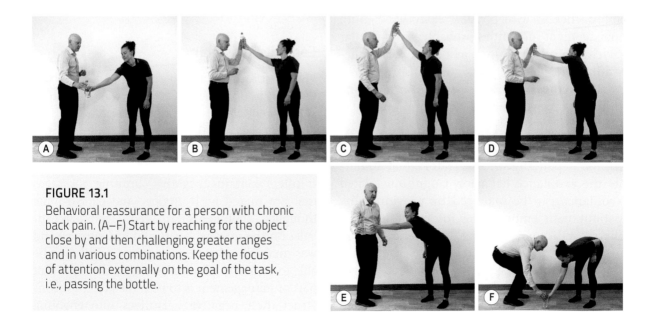

FIGURE 13.1
Behavioral reassurance for a person with chronic back pain. (A–F) Start by reaching for the object close by and then challenging greater ranges and in various combinations. Keep the focus of attention externally on the goal of the task, i.e., passing the bottle.

experience more pain and receive disability support.[53] Similarly, the development of serious back pain disability can be predicted more reliably from the person's psychosocial history than from structural or degenerative changes in the spine.[54]

AVOIDANCE AND REASSURANCE

Beliefs and anxieties about movement may feed a widening gap between an assumed incapacity and the current "potential" physical capacity (Fig. 13.1). This gap tends to widen with conditions that are of longer duration or greater intensity.[55-58] Hence, an important component of the shared management is to narrow this gap by redefining and exploring with the individual what degree of loss is real and what is perceived; this, sometimes, can be tricky to establish.

It was demonstrated in patients with chronic back conditions that pain and functionality can improve as much with cognitive–behavioral approaches as with physical exercise.[59,60] Both management modalities probably share similar psychological processes, associated with alleviating the anxiety, fear, and catastrophizing related to the condition – essentially, conveying the reassuring message that movement is OK.[59,61,62]

Reassurance can be provided in different forms, depending on the factors that underlie the avoidance behavior. Cognition-related avoidance can be managed by providing the patient with empowering information about their condition.[50] Learned, experience-related avoidance can be alleviated by a gradual reintroduction of tasks and movement ranges that the patient has withdrawn from (see graded activity, Chapter 9; demonstration, Chapter 14), as well as cognitive reassurance.[50,63]

Patients who exhibit affective, anxiety-related avoidance may partly respond to behavioral forms of reassurance but may not react well to reasoning or cognitive reassurance. This particular group may benefit from additional psychological care as part of their overall management.[50]

Cognition and behavior are inseparable – a change in cognition relating to the condition will influence the person's recovery behavior. Equally, introducing safe, non-aggravating movement experiences can influence how a person perceives their condition and embolden them to experiment with the movement that they fear (see Fig. 13.1),[63] but usually it is a mixture of both. The outcome from cognitive and behavioral reassurance can be reduced pain, improved movement capacity, a return to more normal occupational and recreational activities, and reduced healthcare-seeking behavior.[28,59,64-67] The bottom line is: it's all about patient empowerment and having a sense of control.

Cognitive reassurance

When an individual experiences pain or movement limitation, they create a personalized story about their condition: how it came about, the nature of the condition, how it will improve, and so on. This internal narrative is derived from numerous sources and previous experiences. It often contains negative, limiting messages that are mixed with anxiety and catastrophic thoughts: "shoulder is damaged – seen torn capsules on the internet – a friend had surgery and was unable to play tennis again – will I ever be able to return to playing tennis?" An important part of management is to help the patient reconstruct their negative narratives into enabling and positive ones.

There are several ways to assist the individual to transform their cognition and narratives. Providing the patient with relevant information about their condition is an important part of this process;[28-30] information that they can do something about, i.e., messages that contain empowering information, is particularly valuable.[68] For example, a dancer suffering from frozen shoulder was given the misinformation that their condition is associated with capsular tears. This resulted in avoidance behavior where the person refrained from using their arm for several months for fear of damaging it. The alternative empowering narrative emphasized the positive aspect of the condition – that the capsule is intact and strong, that it can self-recover, and the condition is unlikely to result in any future disability. Additional information was given about the processes associated with tissue adaptation and how they can be facilitated by daily use of the arm. To disassociate pain from damage, the information included a simplified explanation of the difference between the pain of injury and the pain of sensitization (see Chapter 10). At a session 2 weeks later, the patient exhibited a dramatic increase in shoulder range of movement (ROM) and reported an increase in daily use. The patient attributed this improvement to feeling safe and confident using the arm, even in painful ranges. Generally, the alternative narrative is constructed around empowering messages, such as: "it's safe," "you can do it," "it's uncomplicated," "you have the capacity to recover," and so on.

Focusing on the "abled self", rather than "disabled self," can also be part of cognitive reassurance – pointing out to the patient what they can do, rather than what they cannot. For example, individuals who suffer from chronic back pain can be virtually symptom-free during demanding physical activities such as gardening, playing soccer, or even windsurfing. This could be pointed out during a session, focusing on these "abled"' activities. These messages may be as important as the exercises themselves.

The individual's fears and anxieties may be increased by information which focuses on factors that are outside their control, disempowering information that does not support a return to functionality. Positive information that highlights the central neuromechanisms of persistent pain seems to have a positive effect on pain levels and functionality:[69] essentially, information that disassociates pain from injury and danger. There is questionable, and potentially negative, therapeutic value in providing a detailed description of underlying damage or pathology, and in using pathological anatomical or mechanical models to explain the condition.[70,71] The use of disempowering terms such as "deterioration" or "degeneration" is likely to increase anxiety and avoidance. Even necessary negative information about the condition can be sandwiched between empowering messages. For example, a person with meniscus or disk damage can be told that it is prevalent, even in asymptomatic individuals, that the body has the capacity to recover from this condition, and that being active is helpful. The caveat here is not to create unrealistic expectations for the patient: reassurance has to represent the expected outcome. It is a fine balance, which I am still refining after 36 years in practice!

Behavioral reassurance

Behavioral reassurance aims to minimize avoidance by creating positive physical experiences and narratives in relation to the feared activities.[63-66,72] It involves "movement experiments," in which the individual can reassess what is real and what is assumed loss, and how it impacts their functionality. A useful clinical tool to re-evaluate these preconceptions is the graded challenge described in Chapter 9. These movement challenges can be initiated in the clinic under the supervision and support of the therapist. They are performed within functional tasks using tolerable ranges, often amplifying the four task parameters (force, endurance, ROM, and velocity). For example, in the first session working with individuals who suffer from persistent back pain, I stand facing the patient and ask them to repeatedly pass to me and then retrieve a bottle of water (see Fig. 13.1A–F). During the activity, I keep changing my arm position, holding it progressively further away, and encouraging them to bend in ranges which they may consider to be unsafe. (I have done this for several decades without any mishaps, yet.) This behavioral reassurance is then supplemented by cognitive reassurance; it is brought to the patient's awareness how successful and safe they are in performing these demanding activities.

Can unsuitable exercise convey the wrong message? An unsuitable exercise is one which does not serve the individual's goal of rehabilitation and may conversely increase their condition-related fears through an implicit negative message. For example, it is common to prescribe a supposedly "safe" trunk-strengthening exercise to alleviate or prevent back pain (although it is well established that trunk muscle or core strength is not associated with spinal pain or injury).[73,74] This instruction often comes with advice to limit trunk exertion during daily activities, such as "be careful how you twist and bend" and "don't lift and carry shopping." The implicit negative message here is that daily activities are unsafe and are to be feared; that the spine is weak and needs to be mollycoddled;

that only through the special back exercise is recovery possible. It is not unusual for patients with back pain to turn up in my clinic complaining that their lack of improvement is due to persistently weak spinal or "core" muscles. They often assume that it is brought about by their own failure to perform the exercise correctly or regularly (see guilt and inadequacy below). In these situations, I steer patients towards a functional engagement and away from the specific back exercise, shifting the locus of recovery to the functional domain.

Reassurance for the prescriber

A common clinical concern for the therapist is the safety of the prescribed activities. Will they cause harm? Will the patient sue me? Will I lose my license to practice? The therapist's anxieties could also feed the gap between the real and the assumed damage or deficit. This anxiety is partly associated with assessment and diagnostic uncertainties. Even a simple test such as a ROM examination can be misleading. It is often affected by the patient's fear of pain or re-injury, or by the simple fact that physical examinations can be low on validity and reliability.[75–82] Hence, estimating the actual level of damage can remain unresolved and there is always the possibility that the patient's fears may represent real, safety-related limitations. Added to this is the uncertainty of how the patient will respond to the prescribed activities. These uncertainties could erode the therapist's own confidence in the safety of the treatment and negatively influence management: for example, by prescribing low-intensity, ineffective exercise or unnecessarily limiting the individual's functional repertoire. These apprehensions could feed back to the patient to reinforce their negative beliefs, fears, and avoidance behavior.[37] So, therapists also need reassurance. One solution is to accept uncertainty and plan a management program that accounts for the unknown, primarily by using the graded challenge as discussed in Chapter 9. This can help reassure both the therapist and the patient that movement is safe.

PSYCHOLOGICAL DISTRESS: ROLE OF THE THERAPIST

Injury, pain, and loss of functionality are often associated with natural emotions such as disappointment, anger, frustration, grief, helplessness, hopelessness, and depression. The individual may feel that their body has let them down. These feelings are often accompanied by a change in body and self-image and a deep sense of loss when they are unable to return to their "true" active self.[8]

How we interact with the patient, the therapeutic relationship, can have an important role in alleviating the psychological distress associated with the condition and in supporting the patient in their return to functionality.[29,61,83] Clinical attitudes that include being attentive to the patient's emotional state, displaying empathy, and being non-judgmental, caring, supportive, and encouraging should be the bedrock of the management. For example, the practitioner's empathic presence has been shown to reduce chronic pain substantially over a period of several months.[84] The practitioner's non-verbal communication can also impact the management outcome. Patients are more expressive when their practitioner uses a forward-leaning posture, smiles, nods, and speaks in a relatively high-pitched voice (not much hope for me, being a 62-year-old male with a deep voice). So, what we say and how we interact with the patient can support what we prescribe.[85]

The five horsemen of the exercise apocalypse

Unrealistic and inflexible management may evoke negative feelings that could put the individual off engaging in the prescribed activities, in particular:

- **Guilt** – not doing my exercises since the last session
- **Shame** – telling my therapist or peers about this
- **Embarrassment** – being exposed as being "weak" or "unreliable"
- **Hopelessness** – too many or complex exercises, not enough time in the day to exercise
- **Inadequacy** – can't control my core, unable to learn or remember simple exercise.

These difficult feelings can be minimized by the clinical attitudes described above, as well as by loosely applying the good old SMART principles in the management:

- The prescribed exercises are *specific* to the individual and their condition, and organized within the unique context of their life.
- Their progress is readily *measurable* using, for example, simple 0–10 symptomatic and functional scales that the patient can consult to track their own progress.
- The remedial activities should be *attainable*: uncomplicated and easily implemented within the individual's functional repertoire and capacity.
- The management should be *realistic*, taking into account the individual's life's circumstances.
- The management should be contained within reasonable *time frames*.

Chapter 13

References

1. Anderson CL, Feldman DB. Hope and physical exercise: the contributions of hope, self-efficacy, and optimism in accounting for variance in exercise frequency. Psychol Rep. 2020;123:1145–59.

2. Rhodes RE, de Bruijn GJ. What predicts intention-behavior discordance? A review of the action control framework. Exerc Sport Sci Rev. 2013;41:201–7.

3. Rhodes RE, Yao CA. Models accounting for intention-behavior discordance in the physical activity domain: a user's guide, content overview, and review of current evidence. Int J Behav Nutr Phys Act. 2015;12:9.

4. Holden MA, Haywood KL, Potia TA, Gee M, McLean S. Recommendations for exercise adherence measures in musculoskeletal settings: a systematic review and consensus meeting (protocol). Syst Rev. 2014;3:10.

5. Trost SG, Owen N, Bauman AE, Sallis JF, Brown W. Correlates of adults' participation in physical activity: review and update. Med Sci Sports Exerc. 2002;34:1996–2001.

6. Jordan JL, Holden MA, Mason EE, Foster NE. Interventions to improve adherence to exercise for chronic musculoskeletal pain in adults. Cochrane Database Syst Rev. 2010 Jan 20;1:CD005956.

7. Jack K, McLean SM, Moffett JK, Gardiner E. Barriers to treatment adherence in physiotherapy outpatient clinics: a systematic review. Man Ther. 2010;15:220–8.

8. Smith BE, Hendrick P, Smith TO, Bateman M, Moffatt F, Rathleff MS, et al. Should exercises be painful in the management of chronic musculoskeletal pain? A systematic review and meta-analysis. Br J Sports Med. 2017;51:1679–87.

9. Herring MP, Sailors MH, Bray MS. Genetic factors in exercise adoption, adherence and obesity. Obes Rev. 2014;15:29–39.

10. Chan DK, Lonsdale C, Ho PY, Yung PS, Chan KM. Patient motivation and adherence to postsurgery rehabilitation exercise recommendations: the influence of physiotherapists' autonomy-supportive behaviors. Arch Phys Med Rehabil. 2009;90:1977–82.

11. Jolly K, Taylor R, Lip GY, Greenfield S, Raftery J, Mant J, et al. The Birmingham Rehabilitation Uptake Maximization Study (BRUM). Home-based compared with hospital-based cardiac rehabilitation in a multi-ethnic population: cost-effectiveness and patient adherence. Health Technol Assess. 2007;11:1–118.

12. Sluijs EM, Kok GJ, van der Zee J. Correlates of exercise compliance in physical therapy. Phys Ther. 1993;73:771–82.

13. Duda JL, Smart AE, Tappe MK. Predictors of adherence in the rehabilitation of athletic injuries: an application of personal investment theory. J Sport Exerc Psychol. 1989;11:367–81.

14. Picorelli AM, Pereira LS, Pereira DS, Felício D, Sherrington C. Adherence to exercise programs for older people is influenced by program characteristics and personal factors: a systematic review. J Physiother. 2014;60:151–6.

15. Pérusse L, Tremblay A, Leblanc C, Bouchard C. Genetic and environmental influences on level of habitual physical activity and exercise participation. Am J Epidemiol. 1989;129:1012–22.

16. De Geus E, Bartels M, Kaprio J, Lightfoot J, Thomis M. Genetics of regular exercise and sedentary behaviors. Twin Res Hum Genet. 2014;17:262–71.

17. de Vilhena e Santos DM, Katzmarzyk PT, Teixeira Seabra AF, Ribeiro Maia JA. Genetics of physical activity and physical inactivity in humans. Behav Genet. 2012;42:559–78.

18. Beunen G, Thomis M. Genetic determinants of sports participation and daily physical activity. Int J Obes Relat Metab Disord. 1999;23 Suppl 3:S55–63.

19. Pereira S, Katzmarzyk PT, Gomes TN, Elston R, Maia J. How consistent are genetic factors in explaining leisure-time physical activity and sport participation? The Portuguese Healthy Families Study. Twin Res Hum Genet. 2018;21:369–77.

20. Moran M, Van Cauwenberg J, Hercky-Linnewiel R, Cerin E, Deforche B, Plaut P. Understanding the relationships between the physical environment and physical activity in older adults: a systematic review of qualitative studies. Int J Behav Nutr Phys Act. 2014;11:79.

21. World Health Organization. Adherence to long-term therapies: evidence for action. World Health Organization, 2003.

22. Meade LB, Bearne LM, Sweeney LH, Alageel SH, Godfrey EL. Behaviour change techniques associated with adherence to prescribed exercise in patients with persistent musculoskeletal pain: systematic review. Br J Health Psychol. 2019;24:10–30.

23. Marley J, Tully MA, Porter-Armstrong A, Bunting B, O'Hanlon J, Atkins L, et al. The effectiveness of interventions aimed at increasing physical activity in adults with persistent musculoskeletal pain: a systematic review and meta-analysis. BMC Musculoskelet Disord. 2017;18:1–20.

24. Evenson K, Fleury J. Barriers to outpatient cardiac rehabilitation participation and adherence. J Cardiopulm Rehab. 2000;20:241–6.

25. Locke EA. Toward a theory of task motivation incentives. J Organ Behav Hum Perform. 1966;3:157–89.

26. McCall LA, Ginis KAM. The effects of message framing on exercise adherence and health beliefs among patients in a cardiac rehabilitation program. J Appl Biobehav Res. 2004;9:122–35.

27. Henrotin YE, Cedraschi C, Duplan B, Bazin T, Duquesnoy B. Information and low back pain management: a systematic review. Spine (Phila Pa 1976). 2006;31:E326–34.

28. Burton AK, Waddell, G, Tillotson KM, Summerton N. Information and advice to patients with back pain can have a positive effect. A randomised controlled trial of a novel educational booklet in primary care. Spine. 1999;24:2484–91.

29. Linton SJ, Andersson T. Can chronic disability be prevented? A randomized trial of a cognitive-behavior intervention and two forms of information for patients with spinal pain. Spine. 2000;25:2825–31.

30. Moseley GL, Nicholas MK, Hodges PW. A randomized controlled trial of intensive neurophysiology education in chronic low back pain. Clin J Pain. 2004;20:324–30.

31. Pfingsten M. Functional restoration: it depends on an adequate mixture of treatment. Schmerz. 2001;15:492–8.

32. Jackson L, Leclerc J, Erskine Y, Linden W. Getting the most out of cardiac rehabilitation: a review of referral and adherence predictors. Heart. 2005;91:10–14.

33. Hassett LM, Tate RL, Moseley AM, Gillett LE. Injury severity, age and pre-injury exercise history predict adherence to a home-based exercise programme in adults with traumatic brain injury. Brain Inj. 2011;25:698–706.

34. Dolan-Mullen P, Green LW, Persinger GS. Clinical trials of patient education for chronic conditions: a comparative meta-analysis of intervention types. Prev Med. 1985;14:753–81.

35. Ice R. Long term compliance. Phys Ther. 1985;65:1832–9.

36. Kori S, Miller R, Todd D. Kinesiophobia: a new view of chronic pain behaviour. Pain Man. 1990;3:35–43.

37. Poiraudeau S, Rannou F, Baron G, Henanff LE, Coudyre E, Rozenberg S, et al. Fear-avoidance beliefs about back pain in patients with subacute low back pain. Pain. 2006;124:305–11.

38. Leeuw M, Goossens MEJB, Linton SJ, Crombez G, Boersma K, Vlaeyen JWS. The fear-avoidance model of musculoskeletal pain: current state of scientific evidence. J Behav Med. 2007;30:77–94.

39. Shaw WS, Pransky G, Patterson W, Linton SJ, Winters T. Patient clusters in acute, work-related back pain based on patterns of disability risk factors. J Occup Environ Med. 2007;49:185–93.

40. Elfving B, Andersson T, Grooten WJ. Low levels of physical activity in back pain patients are associated with high levels of fear-avoidance beliefs and pain catastrophizing. Physiother Res Int. 2007;12:14–24.

41. Thomas JS, France CR. Pain-related fear is associated with avoidance of spinal motion during recovery from low back pain. Spine (Phila Pa 1976). 2007;32:E460–6.

42. Thomas JS, France CR, Lavender SA, Johnson MR. Effects of fear of movement on spine velocity and acceleration after recovery from low back pain. Spine (Phila Pa 1976). 2008;33:564–70.

43. George SZ, Wittmer VT, Fillingim RB, Robinson ME. Fear-avoidance beliefs and temporal summation of evoked thermal pain influence self-report of disability in patients with chronic low back pain. J Occup Rehab. 2006;16:95–108.

44. Severeijns R, Vlaeyen JW, van den Hout MA, Weber WE. Pain catastrophizing predicts

pain intensity, disability, and psychological distress independent of the level of physical impairment. Clin J Pain. 2001;17:165–72.

45. Woby SR, Watson PJ, Roach NK, Urmston M. Adjustment to chronic low back pain: the relative influence of fear-avoidance beliefs, catastrophising, and appraisals of control. Behav Res Ther. 2004;42:761–74.

46. Swinkels-Meewisse IE, Roelofs J, Oostendorp RA, Verbeek ALM, Vlaeyen JWS. Acute low back pain: pain-related fear and pain catastrophizing influence physical performance and perceived disability. Pain. 2006;120:36–43.

47. Al-Obaidi SM, Nelson RM, Al-Awadhi S, Al-Shuwaie N. The role of anticipation and fear of pain in the persistence of avoidance behavior in patients with chronic low back pain. Spine. 2000;25:1126–31.

48. Kvist J, Ek A, Sporrstedt K, Good L. Fear of re-injury: a hindrance for returning to sports after anterior cruciate ligament reconstruction. Knee Surg Sports Traumatol Arthrosc. 2005;13:393–7.

49. Crombez G, Vlaeyen JW, Heuts PH, Lysens R. Pain-related fear is more disabling than pain itself: evidence on the role of pain-related fear in chronic back pain disability. Pain. 1999;80:329–39.

50. Rainville J, Smeets RJ, Bendix T, Tveito TH, Poiraudeau S, Indahl AJ, et al. Fear-avoidance beliefs and pain avoidance in low back pain: translating research into clinical practice. Spine J. 2011;11:895–903.

51. Wenzel HG, Vasseljen O, Mykletun A, Nilsen TI. Pre-injury health-related factors in relation to self-reported whiplash: longitudinal data from the HUNT study, Norway. Eur Spine J. 2012;21:1528–35.

52. Kamper SJ, Maher CG, Menezes Costa L da C, McAuley JH, Hush JM, Sterling M. Does fear of movement mediate the relationship between pain intensity and disability in patients following whiplash injury? A prospective longitudinal study. Pain. 2012;153:113–19.

53. Mykletun A, Glozier N, Wenzel HG, Overland S, Harvey SB, Wessely S, et al. Reverse causality in the association between whiplash and symptoms of anxiety and depression: the HUNT study. Spine (Phila Pa 1976). 2011;36:1380–6.

54. Carragee E, Alamin TF, Miller JF, Carragee JM. Discographic, MRI and psychosocial determinants of low back pain disability and remission: a prospective study in subjects with benign persistent back pain. Spine J. 2005;5:24–35.

55. Grotle M, Vøllestad NK, Veierød MB, Brox JI. Fear-avoidance beliefs and distress in relation to disability in acute and chronic low back pain. Pain. 2004;112:343–52.

56. Grotle M, Vøllestad NK, Brox JI. Clinical course and impact of fear-avoidance beliefs in low back pain: prospective cohort study of acute and chronic low back pain: II. Spine (Phila Pa 1976). 2006;31:1038–46.

57. Pincus T, Vogel S, Burton AK, Santos R, Field AP. Fear avoidance and prognosis in back pain: a systematic review and synthesis of current evidence. Arthritis Rheum. 2006;54:3999–4010.

58. Vangronsveld K, Peters M, Goossens M, Vlaeyen J. The influence of movement and pain catastrophising on daily pain and disability in individuals with acute whiplash injury: a daily diary study. Pain. 2008;139:449–57.

59. Smeets RJ, Vlaeyen JW, Kester AD, Knottnerus JA. Reduction of pain catastrophizing mediates the outcome of both physical and cognitive-behavioral treatment in chronic low back pain. J Pain. 2006;7:261–71.

60. Critchley DJ, Ratcliffe J, Noonan S, Jones RH, Hurley MV. Effectiveness and cost-effectiveness of three types of physiotherapy used to reduce chronic low back pain disability: a pragmatic randomized trial with economic evaluation. Spine. 2007;32:1474–8.

61. Ikemoto T, Miki K, Matsubara T, Wakao N. Psychological treatment strategy for chronic low back pain. Spine Surg Relat Res. 2018;3:199–206.

62. Steptoe A, Edwards S, Moses J, Mathews A. The effects of exercise training on mood and perceived coping ability in anxious adults from the general population. J Psychosom Res. 1989;33:537 47.

63. Vlaeyen JW, Linton SJ. Fear-avoidance model of chronic musculoskeletal pain: 12 years on. Pain. 2012;153:1144–7.

64. Linton SJ, Ryberg M. A cognitive-behavioral group

intervention as prevention for persistent neck and back pain in a non-patient population: a randomized controlled trial. Pain. 2001;90:83–90.

65. Linton SJ, Boersma K, Jansson M, Svärd L, Botvalde M. The effects of cognitive-behavioral and physical therapy preventive interventions on pain-related sick leave: a randomized controlled trial. Clin J Pain. 2005;21:109–19.

66. Linton SJ, Nordin E. A 5-year follow-up evaluation of the health and economic consequences of an early cognitive behavioral intervention for back pain: a randomized, controlled trial. Spine. 2006;31:853–8.

67. Hoffman BM, Papas RK, Chatkoff DK, Kerns RD. Meta-analysis of psychological interventions for chronic low back pain. Health Psychol. 2007;26:1–9.

68. Crow R, Gage H, Hampson S, Hart J, Kimber A, Thomas H. The role of expectancies in the placebo effect and their use in the delivery of health care: a systematic review. Health Technol Assess. 1999;3:1–96.

69. Marris D, Theophanous K, Cabezon P, Dunlap Z, Donaldson M. The impact of combining pain education strategies with physical therapy interventions for patients with chronic pain: a systematic review and meta-analysis of randomized controlled trials. Physiother Theory Pract. 2019;30:1–2.

70. Louw A, Diener I, Butler DS, Puentedura EJ. The effect of neuroscience education on pain, disability, anxiety, and stress in chronic musculoskeletal pain. Arch Phys Med Rehabil. 2011;92: 2041–56.

71. Werner EL, Storheim K, Løchting I, Wisløff T, Grotle M. Cognitive patient education for low back pain in primary care: a cluster randomized controlled trial and cost-effectiveness analysis. Spine (Phila Pa 1976). 2016;41:455–62.

72. Linton SJ, Boersma K, Jansson M, Overmeer T, Lindblom K, Vlaeyen JWS. A randomized controlled trial of exposure in vivo for patients with spinal pain reporting fear of work-related activities. Eur J Pain. 2008;12:722–30.

73. Hamberg-van Reenen HH. Systematic review of the relation between physical capacity and future low back and neck/shoulder pain. Pain. 2007;130:93–107.

74. Lederman E. The myth of core stability. J Bodyw Mov Ther. 2010;14:84–98.

75. Paulet T, Fryer G. Inter-examiner reliability of palpation for tissue texture abnormality in the thoracic paraspinal region. IJOM 2009;1:92–6.

76. May S, Littlewood C, Bishop A. Reliability of procedures used in the physical examination of non-specific low back pain: a systematic review. Aust J Physiother. 2006;52:91–102.

77. van Trijffel E, Anderegg Q, Bossuyt PM, Lucas C. Inter-examiner reliability of passive assessment of intervertebral motion in the cervical and lumbar spine: a systematic review. Man Ther. 2005;10:256–69.

78. Seffinger MA, Najm WI, Mishra SI, Adams A, Dickerson VM, Murphy LS, et al. Reliability of spinal palpation for diagnosis of back and neck pain: a systematic review of the literature. Spine (Phila Pa). 2004;29: E413–25.

79. Dunk NM, Chung YY, Compton DS, Callaghan JP. The reliability of quantifying upright standing postures as a baseline diagnostic clinical tool. J Manipulative Physiol Ther. 2004;27:91–6.

80. Hollerwöger D. Methodological quality and outcomes of studies addressing manual cervical spine examinations: a review. Man Ther. 2006; 11:93–8.

81. McCaw ST, Bates BT. Biomechanical implications of mild leg length inequality. Br J Sports Med. 1991;25:10–13.

82. Mannello DM. Leg length inequality. J Manipulative Physiol Ther. 1992;15:576–90.

83. Bieber C, Müller KG, Blumenstiel K, Schneider A, Richter A, Wilke S, et al. Long-term effects of a shared decision-making intervention on physician-patient interaction and outcome in fibromyalgia. A qualitative and quantitative 1 year follow-up of a randomized controlled trial. Patient Educ Couns. 2006;63:357–66.

84. Cánovas L, Carrascosa AJ, García M, Fernández M, Calvo A, Monsalve V, et al. Impact of empathy in the patient-doctor relationship on chronic pain relief and quality of life: a prospective study in

spanish pain clinics. Pain Med. 2018;19:1304–14.

85. Miciak M, Gross DP, Joyce A. A review of the psychotherapeutic 'common factors' model and its application in physical therapy: the need to consider general effects in physical therapy practice. Scand J Caring Sci. 2012;26:394–403.

86. Náfrádi L, Kostova Z, Nakamoto K, Schulz PJ. The doctor-patient relationship and patient resilience in chronic pain: a qualitative approach to patients' perspectives. Chronic Illn. 2018;14:256–70.

87. Kiesler DJ, Auerbach SM. Integrating measurement of control and affiliation in studies of physician-patient interaction: the interpersonal circumplex. Soc Sci Med. 2003;57:1707–22.

Chapter 14

Contents
Summary: constructing a functional exercise management program

Presumably you have reached this point in the book wondering how to put everything together into a coherent and effective exercise prescription plan. This chapter demonstrates how to construct exercise management for some of the more common musculoskeletal and pain conditions that I regularly see in my clinic. It will focus on exercise prescription for recovering activities associated with the shared repertoire (activities of daily living). Examples of exercise prescription for sports rehabilitation have been discussed elsewhere in the book, particularly in Chapter 9. The basic

principle is that all sports activities can become remedial simply by attenuating or amplifying the activity. In clinic, I rarely give an athlete extra-functional exercise. The management is constructed around their particular sporting activity.

How, then, do we construct a functional and process approach-based exercise prescription? The first step is to *identify the process by which the individual will recover from their condition*. Most musculoskeletal conditions are likely to fall into one or combination of these groups:

Condition	All acute conditions and flareups within the expected timeframe of repair, e.g.:	All conditions affecting functional capacity and control of performance (not necessarily associated with repair or pain), e.g.:	All conditions where symptoms persist beyond the expected duration of repair, e.g.:
	All acute tissue damage Acute pain, whether with or without injury Joint and muscle sprains Acute low back and neck pain, including disk-related conditions Immediate period post-surgery Blunt trauma Painful phase of frozen shoulder Acute tendinopathies Acute flareups in persistent pain conditions, e.g., low back and arthritis Overuse injuries?	Conditions affecting task performance Conditions affecting task components (force, endurance, speed and range of movement, balance and coordination) Later, remodeling phase of repair Restorative phase post-surgery Conditions where inducing structural / biomechanical change is recommended for recovery Post-immobilization, detraining ROM loss, e.g., stiff phase of frozen shoulder CNS damage Postural and movement re-education/ rehabilitation	All persistent, pain, discomfort, and stiffness experiences Chronic low back and neck pain Chronic arthritic pain Chronic tendinopathies? Overuse injuries?
Recovery process	Repair	Adaptation	Alleviation of symptoms

Next, the unique features of the exercise management can be worked out from the condition-related recovery process:

Condition	All acute conditions and flareups within the repair time frame	All conditions affecting functional capacity and control of performance	All conditions where symptoms persist beyond the expected duration of repair
Recovery process	**Repair**	**Adaptation**	**Alleviation of symptoms**
Specific management	Cyclical and repetitive loading	**Active movement**	**All forms of exercise; functional may have an advantage over extra-functional**
	Applied locally to affected area	**Functional, task-specific**	
	Initially, movement can be fragmented to specific joints	**Whole and goal movement**	**Discomfort / some pain likely and generally OK, but beware of inducing recurrent flareups**
	Active or passive movement	**Frequent exposure and duration in goal activity**	
	Any movement pattern but preferably functional. Extra-functional is OK but should be rapidly replaced by functional activities	**Discomfort likely and generally OK**	*Activity grading:* **from current functional level and up. No need for attenuation except when used for reassurance (but to be used very sparingly)**
		Activity grading: **from current functional level and up (no need for attenuation)**	
	Tolerable discomfort / pain-free movement		
	Activity grading: initially, may need attenuation to sub-functional intensities and then amplification to low / moderate functional loading		

At this point the overall principles of the activities/exercises are established. Now we need to consider the actual physical form of the exercise. This is partly determined by the location of the condition within the four functional regions: for example:

	Trunk conditions	Leg conditions	Arm conditions	Neck conditions
Consider these activities and exercise from the shared repertoire, e.g.:	All activities	All upright/weight-bearing activities:	Reach and retrieve	All activities
	Bending, twisting	Sit-to-stand	Pull–push	In particular, those requiring head and neck engagement, e.g., turning to look
	Lifting	Stand	Carry	
	Carrying	Walk	Manipulate objects with the hand	
		Use stairs		

These categories enable us to select activities that increase or decrease the physical demands on the affected area (see Chapter 2). Remember that all tasks involve the whole body, so there is a lot of overlap: for example, reaching movements can be used to rehabilitate the shoulder but also a knee or low back condition.

We have now constructed a top-notch personalized and condition-specific exercise management; however, we have to ensure that the individual will actually comply with and adhere to this plan. These participation targets are supported by the features of the shared management (see Chapter 13):

Condition	See above	See above	See above
Recovery process	Repair	Adaptation	Alleviation of symptoms
Specific management	See above	See above	See above
Shared management	Psychological: ease movement/pain-related anxieties and catastrophizing, support, reassure, comfort, soothe and calm		
	Therapeutic relationship: keep professional boundaries, non-judgmental and empathic presence, clear communication, validation of patient's experience, respectful attitude to patient's beliefs		
	Cognitive: inform, involve patient in planning and goal setting, provide choice		
	Behavioral: support recovery behavior, raise awareness of avoidance behavior		
	Keep the remedial activities familiar, integrated within the patient's daily movement repertoire, easily accessible, and uncomplicated		

Once the person has been rehabilitated within their shared repertoire, they can progress to recover their unique group of activities, including sports, using the grading system described in Chapter 9.

We now have an overall structure for developing an exercise plan (Fig. 14.1, over the page).

With this flow chart in mind, we are ready to look at exercise prescription for commonly seen musculoskeletal and pain conditions. Below are some examples of recent patients that I have seen in clinic and the exercise that they were prescribed. Although exercise prescription forms an important part of my overall remedial management, I do use other treatment modalities, such as manual therapy and cognitive–behavioral approaches.

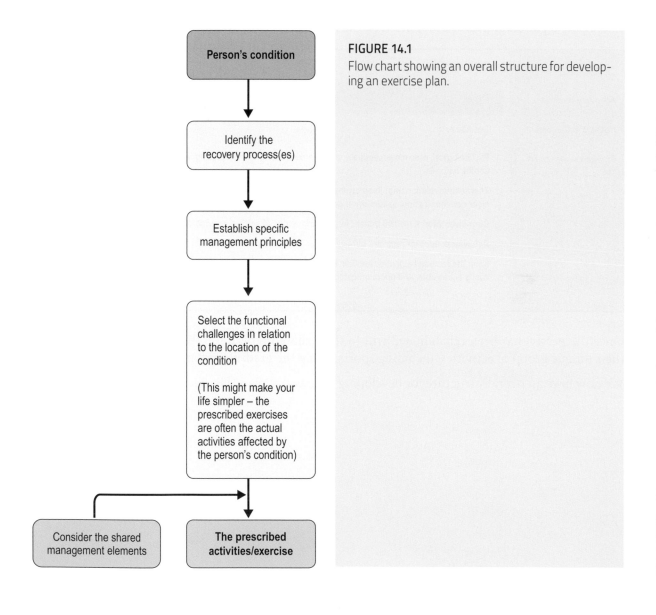

FIGURE 14.1
Flow chart showing an overall structure for developing an exercise plan.

Person's condition

Identify the recovery process(es)

Establish specific management principles

Select the functional challenges in relation to the location of the condition

(This might make your life simpler – the prescribed exercises are often the actual activities affected by the person's condition)

Consider the shared management elements

The prescribed activities/exercise

ACUTE NON-SPECIFIC LOW BACK PAIN

Patient's condition	Acute non-specific low back pain
Recovery process	Repair
Feature of activities/exercise	Cyclical and repetitive loading
	Applied locally to the trunk
	Tolerable discomfort/pain-free movement
	Active or passive movement
	Any movement pattern but preferably functional
	Extra-functional is OK but should be rapidly replaced by functional activities
	Activity grading: initially, may need attenuation but maintain low/moderate functional loading
Consider prescribing these functional activities	All activities can be used "but let pain guide you"
	During the protective phase, keep active, e.g., frequent short walks several times a day
	At the restorative phase, sports and other unique activities can be gradually reintroduced (roughly when pain levels fall to below 4/10). For sports-specific rehabilitation see Chapter 9
Management considerations	Explain pain of injury
	"No need for special back exercise; just walk it off"
	Reassure patient that, with good management, acute back pain resolves rapidly, often within 1–3 weeks

ACUTE LUMBAR DISK WITH/WITHOUT RADICULAR INVOLVEMENT

Patient's condition	Acute lumbar disk with/without radicular involvement
Recovery process	Repair
Feature of activities/exercise	Cyclical and repetitive loading
	Involving the trunk
	Tolerable discomfort/pain-free movement
	Active or passive movement
	Any movement pattern but preferably functional
	Extra-functional is OK but should be rapidly replaced by functional activities
	Activity grading: initially, may need attenuation but maintain low/moderate functional loading by maintaining daily activities
Consider prescribing these functional activities	All activities can be used "but let pain guide you"
	During the protective phase, keep active, especially by walking, e.g., frequent short walks several times a day
	At the restorative phase, sports and other unique activities can be gradually reintroduced (roughly when pain levels fall to below 4/10)
Management considerations	Explain pain of injury and demystify the disk. "You have sprained your back. The disk, like any other joint in the body, will recover through repair. Pain and leg symptoms are likely to recover as the area heals. Movement is a great healer; keep on moving." "No need for special back exercise; just walk it off"
	Reassure the patient that, with good management, acute disk conditions can resolve within 4–8 weeks

Note: Patients with acute lower back pain may experience small benefits in pain relief and functional improvement if given advice to stay active, as opposed to advice to rest in bed. Patients with sciatica experience little or no difference between the two approaches.[1] However, there are potential harmful effects with prolonged rest; therefore, stay active. Additionally, there seems to be no difference between exercising (extra-functional) and staying active (functional).[1] So, keep it simple and functional.

CHRONIC NON-SPECIFIC LOW BACK PAIN

Patient's condition	Chronic non-specific low back pain
Recovery process	Alleviation of symptoms
Feature of activities/exercise	Any movement pattern but preferably functional
	Tolerable discomfort/pain during the exercise session and for short duration afterwards is OK
	Frequent exposure to the activity during the day (e.g., three walks per day may be better than one long one)
	Activity grading: from current capacity and up towards full functional engagement, particularly for those who have withdrawn from activities due to pain and movement-related anxieties
Consider prescribing these functional activities	All functional and extra-functional activities can be used
	Walking: increase distance and pace
	Bend and lift: pick objects up from the floor by bending from standing rather than squatting (Fig. 14.2A–E)
	Bending and twisting, e.g., repetitions of loading the dishwasher or tying shoelaces while standing and bending rather than squatting
	Carrying, e.g., light shopping, alternating one bag between hands or two bags in both hands, progressively increasing the weight (Fig. 14.3A–D)
Management considerations	Explain pain of sensitivity. Spine is not damaged, just sensitive. The structural strength is no different to that in a pain-free individual – hence, safe to resume the full functional repertoire, including sports activities
	The management is more about reassurance and functionality (see Chapter 13)

Note: Remember that functional recovery can come about by reducing pain but also by alleviating movement-related anxieties. Advise the patient to use the back and bend it during daily activities, including ordinary lifting; this is safe and beneficial.[2]
No need to limit physical activities.[3]
Lifting with straight legs and bent spine is not bad for your back.[4]
Lifting loads over 25 kg and lifting at a frequency of over 25 lifts/day increase the annual incidence of low back pain by about 4%.[5]

FROZEN SHOULDER: PAINFUL PHASE

Frozen shoulder is a disorder that is initially marked by inflammation in the glenohumeral joint.[6] It is not associated with loss of tissue tensile strength: it is not an injury (although rarely it can be caused by trauma to the upper body). The aim in this condition is to help resolve the painful stage with movement.

Patient's condition	Painful frozen shoulder
Recovery process	Repair (i.e., resolution of inflammation)
Feature of activities/exercise	High-repetition, cyclical movement
	Can be done several times a day to control pain
	Applied locally to the shoulder
	Pain-free movement ranges
	Active or passive movement
	Any movement pattern but preferably functional
	Activity grading: initially, likely to be attenuated due to intensity of pain. Often, there is marked protection behavior of the arm. It may take a few weeks to subside and be replaced by restorative behavior. Functional engagement should be encouraged along with these improvements
Consider prescribing these functional activities	Walking (or standing), introducing arm swings in flexion–extension cycles (often least painful). Add adduction–abduction in front and back of the trunk as condition permits. Later, as pain-free range improves, add internal–external rotation by sticking elbows out while swinging the arm in flexion–extension cycles (Fig. 14.4A–G)
	Initially, if the patient is in too much pain to perform active swings, these movements can be introduced as passive movement by the therapist
Management considerations	Explain to the patient the nature of the condition and how the shoulder is fully intact. It is as strong as the other non-painful side and any flareup is due to pain sensitivity caused by inflammation rather than re-injury
	Don't stretch the painful shoulder – it's pain from hell and will really make it angry![7]
	This management can reduce the painful phase from many months to about 4–8 weeks only

FROZEN SHOULDER: STIFF PHASE

In the stiff phase, inflammation and pain are mostly resolved but the person is left with severe movement restrictions due to excessive fibrosis, contracture, and thickening of the shoulder's capsule, ligaments, and tendons: in particular, the anterior aspect of the capsule, coracohumeral ligament, and biceps tendon (adhesions are not commonly found).[8-10]

Patient's condition	Frozen shoulder: stiff phase
Recovery process	Adaptation
Feature of activities/exercise	Functional, whole-task activities
	Frequent repetition throughout the day
	Activity grading: amplify from sub-functional to functional level
	Focus on all task parameters, in particular the range component[11]
Consider prescribing these functional activities	All reaching, lifting, and carrying tasks. Note that the shoulder is intact so any force can be used safely (Figs 14.5A–C, 14.6A–F, 14.7A–B, and 14.8A–H)
	May need therapist's help initially (Fig. 14.9A–H)
Management considerations	Explain biomechanical stiffness (see Chapter 12) and training conditions for adaptation – specificity (using exercises that resemble daily activities), need for high-volume exposure and overloading (training above the current capacity) (see Chapter 7)
	Highlight that the current remaining pain is due to sensitivity, not damage or inflammation, and that the structural strength is no different from that of the unaffected side – hence, it is safe to resume the full functional repertoire, ideally at end-ranges where an uncomfortable stretch is experienced (Fig. 14.5A–C)

POST-OPERATIVE SHOULDER: ACUTE EARLY PHASE

Patient's condition	Post-operative shoulder: immediate early protective phase
Recovery process	Repair (inflammation and proliferation phases)
Feature of activities/exercise	**Always follow the surgeon's recommendations; if unsure, consult with them** Cyclical, repetitive movement Can be done several times a day to control pain Applied locally to the shoulder Pain-free movement ranges Active or passive movement Functional or extra-functional Activity grading: initially, attenuated movement according to guidelines.
Consider prescribing these functional activities	Low-amplitude/force, cyclical flexion–extension or rotation cycles can be performed in a sling or supported with the other arm (Figs 14.10A–F and 14.11A–C). With improvement, these can be replaced by unsupported pendulum swings (Fig. 14.4A–G)
Management considerations	"Let pain (and the surgeon) guide you"

POST-OPERATIVE SHOULDER: REMODELING AND RESTORATIVE PHASE

Patient's condition	Post-operative shoulder: remodeling and restorative phase
Recovery process	Adaptation (remodeling phase)
Feature of activities/exercise	**Always follow the surgeon's recommendations; if unsure consult with them** Functional, whole-task activities Frequent repetition throughout the day Activity grading: amplify from sub-functional to functional level Focus on all task parameters (force, endurance, range, and velocity)
Consider prescribing these functional activities	After surgery it will take several weeks for tissues to regain some of their tensile strength, so the activity grading should start at a low level with tolerable discomfort (Figs 14.9A–F, 14.5A–C, 14.6A–E, 14.7A–B, and 14.8A–H)
Management considerations	"Practice frequently what you aim to recover and the body will follow." Repeat this message to the patient often

Note: Different surgical procedures may require specific restricted movement ranges during the initial phases of rehabilitation, such as limited external rotation. As a safety precaution, clarify with the surgeon what these are before commencing with the exercise plan.

Chapter 14

POST-OPERATIVE OR PAINFUL FLAREUP ARTHRITIC HIP

Patient's condition	Acute hip
Recovery process	Repair (see Chapters 4–5)
Feature of activities/exercise	**Always follow the surgeon's recommendations; if unsure, consult with them** Cyclical, repetitive movement Can be done several times a day to control pain Applied locally to the knee Strive for pain-free movement ranges; some pain may, however, be inevitable Active or passive movement Mostly whole-task rehabilitation, except for a short period in the beginning when management may have to be fragmented, sub- or extra-functional Activity grading: attenuation to amplification. Attenuate whole-task activities in the protective phase; may need crutch for support
Consider prescribing these functional activities	During the early repair period: low-amplitude/force, cyclical flexion–extension cycles can be performed in sitting and standing (Figs 14.12A–B and 14.13A–E) Gradual loading of the affected side by shifting body weight; at one point, introduce small, tolerable bending and straightening the knee with partial and then full weight-bearing. This can be vertically graded by reaching tasks in the direction of the affected side (Fig. 14.14A–E) Step with affected side to a low stair without raising (for hip flexion), then two stairs high. Step with unaffected side as above for extension of the affected side (Fig. 14.15A–B) For managing the restorative phase, see below
Management considerations	"Let pain guide you but some discomfort is inevitable"

POST-OPERATIVE HIP: REMODELING AND RESTORATIVE PHASE

Patient's condition	Post-operative hip, latter restorative phase
Recovery process	Adaptation (remodeling phase)
Feature of activities/exercise	**Always follow the surgeon's recommendations; if unsure, consult with them** Functional, whole-task activities Frequent repetition throughout the day Activity grading: amplify from sub-functional to functional level Focus on all task components: force, endurance, range, velocity, balance and organization duration
Consider prescribing these functional activities	As management enters the latter phase of repair, gradually amplify daily activities. Introduce whole-task rehabilitation and gradual return to daily activities Sit-to-stand (Figs 14.16A–F, 14.17A–C, and 14.18A–B) Walking: increase stride length and speed, then step over obstacles (Fig. 14.19A–B). Walk and turn can be used to challenge hip external–internal rotation (Fig. 14.20A–B). For hip extension, consider challenges in Figure 14.21A–B Stair challenges as in Figures 14.15A–B and 14.22A–C, then stepping on each step with both legs to, eventually, frequent normal use of stairs If postural steadiness is affected, add balance challenges (Figs 14.20A–B, 14.19A–B, and 14.23A–B). Add slow walking, spending more time on the affected side and challenging dynamic balance
Management considerations	"Practice frequently what you aim to recover and the body will follow". Repeat this message to the patient often.

Note: Different surgical procedures may require specific restricted movement ranges during the initial phases of rehabilitation. As a safety precaution, clarify with the surgeon what these are before commencing with the exercise plan.

Chapter 14

ACUTE KNEE INJURIES AND POST SURGERY

This exercise prescription could be suitable for a wide range of knee injuries where conservative management is recommended. This management can be also used for post-surgical rehabilitation.

Patient's condition	Acute knee injury/post-operative
Recovery process	Repair (see Chapters 4–5)
Feature of activities/exercise	**Always follow the surgeon's recommendations; if unsure, consult with them**
	Cyclical, repetitive movement
	Can be done several times a day to control pain
	Applied locally to the knee
	Strive for pain-free movement ranges; some pain may, however, be inevitable
	Active or passive movement
	Mostly whole-task rehabilitation, except for a short period in the beginning when movement may have to be fragmented and practiced at sub- or extra-functional levels
	Activity grading: attenuate whole-task activities in the protective phase; may need crutch for support
Consider prescribing these functional activities	Walking: aided or unaided, depending on the extent of tissue damage
	During the early repair period: low-amplitude/force, cyclical flexion–extension cycles can be performed in standing and – once able to flex to 90° – in sitting on a table or chair (Fig. 14.24A–D)
	Gradual loading of the affected side by shifting body weight; at one point, introduce small, tolerable bending and straightening of the knee with partial and then full weight-bearing. This can be vertically graded by reaching tasks in the direction of the affected side (Fig. 14.14A–E)
	Step with affected side to a low stair without going up (for knee flexion), then two stairs high (Fig. 14.15A–B). For knee extension step up with unaffected side, without going up
	As management enters the latter phase of repair, gradually amplify daily activities, such as sit-to-stand, walking, and using stairs (see Chapter 8)
Management considerations	"Let pain guide you but some discomfort is inevitable"

KNEE POST-SURGERY: REMODELING AND RESTORATIVE PHASE

Patient's condition	Post-surgery knee: remodeling and restorative phase
Recovery process	Adaptation
Feature of activities/exercise	**Always follow the surgeon's recommendations; if unsure, consult with them**
	Functional, whole-task activities
	Frequent repetition throughout the day
	Activity grading: amplify from sub-functional to functional level
	Focus on all task components: force, endurance, range, velocity, balance and organization duration
Consider prescribing these functional activities	Sit-to-stand (Figs 14.16A–F, 14.17A–C, and 14.18A–B)
	Walking: increase stride length and speed, then step over obstacle (Fig. 14.19A–B)
	Amplify activities that challenge extension range (Figs 14.21A–B and 14.15B (stepping up with the *unaffected* side)
	Stair challenges and then stepping on each step with both legs to, eventually, normal stair use (Fig. 14.22A–C)
	If postural steadiness is affected, add balance challenges (Figs 14.20A–B, 14.19A–B, and 14.23A–B)
Management considerations	"Let pain guide you but some pain is inevitable"

ACUTE NON-SPECIFIC NECK PAIN

Patient's condition	Acute non-specific neck pain, whiplash
Recovery process	Repair
Feature of activities/exercise	Cyclical and repetitive loading Involve the neck Tolerable discomfort/pain-free movement Active or passive movement Any movement pattern but preferably functional Activity grading: initially, may need attenuation but maintain low/moderate functional challenges
Consider prescribing these functional activities	All daily activities can be used During the protective phase, keep active, especially by walking, e.g., frequent short walks several times a day. Keep trying to rotate the neck, even in the presence of some pain Use movement within a comfortable range to support repair (Figs 14.25A–D and 14.26A–B) At the restorative phase, sports and other unique activities can be gradually reintroduced (roughly when pain levels fall below 4/10)
Management considerations	Pain of injury explained Reassure that, with good management, most acute neck pain resolves rapidly within 1–3 weeks

CHRONIC NON-SPECIFIC NECK PAIN

Patient's condition	Chronic non-specific neck pain and stiffness
Recovery process	Alleviation of symptoms
Feature of activities/exercise	General non-specific movement
	Any movement pattern but preferably functional
	Intensity can be moderate to high physical activity, including sports
	Tolerable discomfort/pain during the exercise session and for short duration afterwards is OK
	Frequent exposure to the affected activity during the day
	Activity grading: from current capacity and up towards full functional engagement, particularly for those who have withdrawn from activities due to pain and movement-related anxieties
Consider prescribing these functional activities	Walking: increase distance and pace, and swing the arms more (this gives greater counter-rotation between the head and body mass) (Fig. 14.27)
	Full side, twisting, and reaching-back activities – challenge head and neck (Fig. 14.26A–B)
	Rotate to stiff end-range and nod head in yes–yes/no–no head gestures (Fig. 14.25A–D)
	Body scan relaxation: the micro-relaxation. Over the years I have found in my clinic that the body scan relaxation can dramatically improve the symptoms of chronic neck pain, including scapular and dorsal pain. The patient can be taught this method in sitting (or any) position. Starting from the feet, raise awareness of the contact of the feet and their weight on the floor, contact of pelvis with the seat, back with back support: "feel the weight of the arms and shoulders, neck and head; let every part melt/soften, let gravity do its work," etc. (think of soothing and calming). The body scan is about 15–20 seconds long (I call it a *micro-relaxation*), and can be repeated throughout the day when the patient becomes aware of tension and pain in these areas. Improvement is often rapid: I give patients a 3–6-week estimate, even in many cases of chronic persistent neck pain that has been present for months and sometimes years!
Management considerations	Explain pain of sensitivity – "neck is not damaged, just sensitive." The structural strength is no different to that in a pain-free individual, hence, it is safe to resume the full functional repertoire

EXERCISES

On the following pages, examples of prescribed exercises for common musculoskeletal conditions are presented. On the figures, the symbols + to +++++ are used to indicate minimum to maximum effect of the challenge on the task components.

Trunk and spine

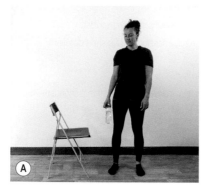 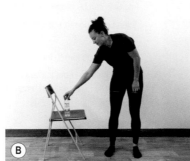 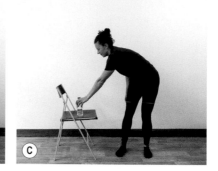

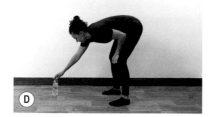 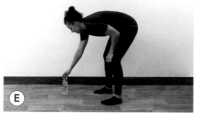

FIGURE 14.2

Description
Grading trunk challenges:
Side-bending (A–B), rotation (C), and flexion (D–E) reaching tasks

Components
Range + to +++++
Endurance + to +++++ by increasing repetition
Force + to +++++ by increasing weight of bottle

Notes
From one session to another, keep challenging the range. Encourage patient to engage in activities that challenge bending from standing rather than squatting or avoiding these activities: loading and clearing dishwasher or loading groceries from floor level to fridge, etc.
These challenges can be used to promote range desensitization as well as for rehabilitation after surgery

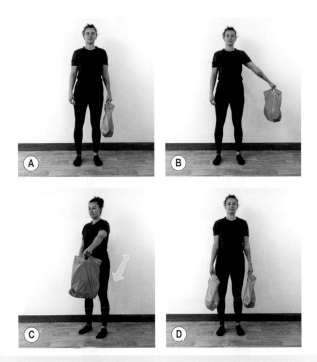

FIGURE 14.3

Description

Loading the trunk/spine by carrying (shopping, briefcase, etc.) One side, keep passing the weight between sides (A) Sustained holding away from the body to the side (B) In sustained flexion or extension or rhythmically swinging the weight while walking (C) Bilateral carrying (D)

Components

Endurance + to +++++ by increasing duration

Force + to +++++ by increasing weight and angle

Notes

Encourage frequent carrying. If shopping with a cart, make it a point to use hand baskets to collect the produce and bring it to the cart

Shoulder and arm

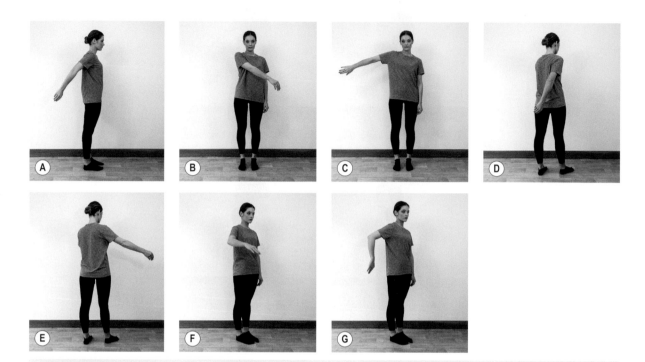

FIGURE 14.4

Description

Supporting repair in shoulder injury/post-surgery after removal of sling

Pendulum swings in various planes:

   Flexion–extension (A)

   Adduction–abduction (B–C)

   Adduction–abduction in extension (behind back) (D–E): ask the patient to stick their elbows out while swinging their arms by the side of their body

   Internal–external rotation (F–G)

Components

Range + to +++ (all ranges of movement)

Notes

In the acute phase the movement should be within the pain-free ranges, gradually increasing in range as pain diminishes

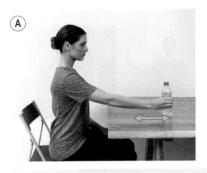 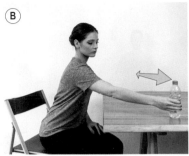 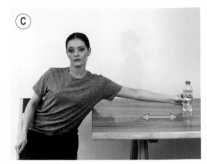

FIGURE 14.5

Description

Shoulder ROM challenges using reaching and retrieving activities

Flexion (A–B)

Increase flexion by increasing distance from table

Abduction–adduction (C)

Components

Range + to +++++

Force + to +++++ by increasing weight

Notes

Start by reaching for object close by and then challenging with greater ranges and in various movement combinations

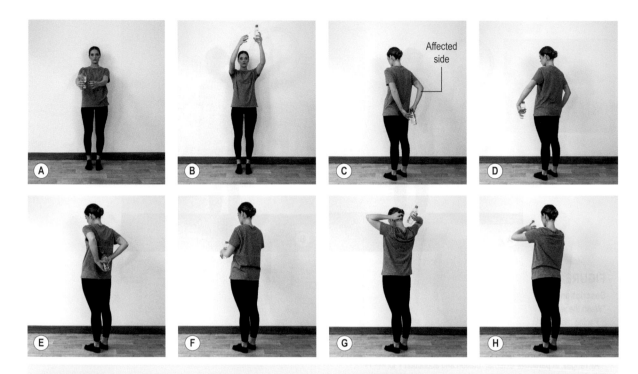

FIGURE 14.8

Description

Pass the bottle/object from one hand to the other at end-ranges:

Flexion (A–B)

Internal rotation. Passing the bottle around the body, low challenge with straight arms behind (C–D)

As above but with arm further up the back (E–F)

External rotation and abduction. Passing the bottle around the head (G–H)

Components

Range + to +++++

Force + to +++ depending on weight

Endurance (dynamic) ++ to +++++

Notes

Any object can be used in this group of challenges

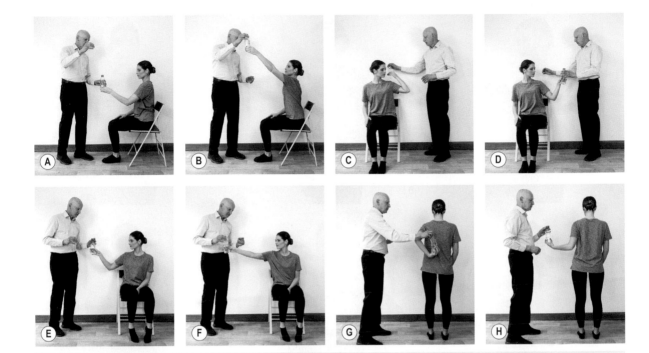

FIGURE 14.9

Description

Therapist leads shoulder ROM challenges:

Flexion range (A–B)

External rotation (C–D)

Abduction–adduction (E–F)

Internal–external rotation (G–H)

Components

Range + to +++++

Endurance + to +++++ by increasing repetition

Force + to +++++ by increasing weight

Notes

Start by reaching for object close by and then challenging with greater ranges and in various combinations

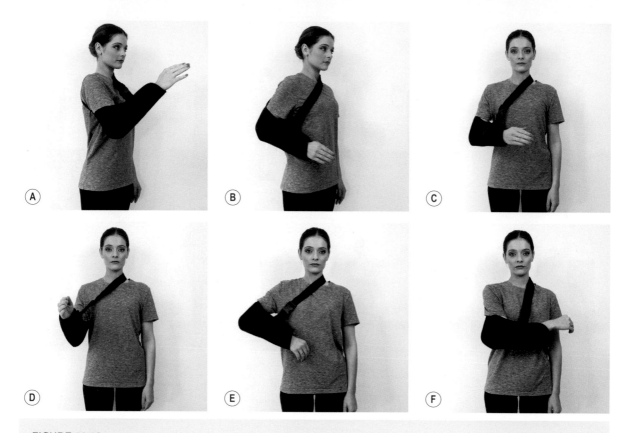

FIGURE 14.10

Description

Support repair in shoulder injury/post-surgery

Cyclical pendulum swings while in sling:

Flexion–extension (A–B)

Internal–external rotation (C–D)

Abduction–adduction (E–F)

Components

Range + to +++ (all ranges)

Notes

All these movements can be integrated into walking. In the acute phase they should be within the pain-free ranges, gradually increasing as range desensitizes

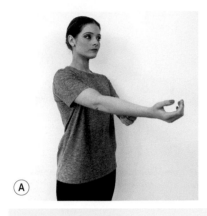
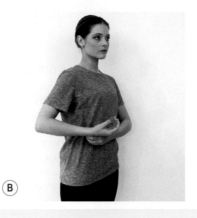
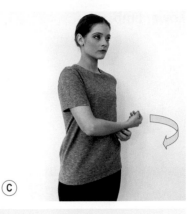

(A)   (B)   (C)

FIGURE 14.11

Description

Supporting repair in shoulder injury/post-surgery after removal of sling

Self-supported cyclical movement:

    Flexion–extension (A–B)

    Internal–external rotation (C)

Components

    Range + to +++ (all ranges of movement)

    Force + to ++

Notes

In the acute phase they should be within the pain-free ranges, gradually increasing as range desensitizes

Lower limb

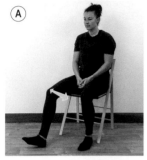

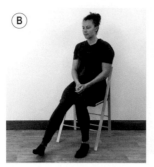

FIGURE 14.12

Description

Low-load, off-weight-bearing hip pendulum movements during sitting
  Adduction–abduction and external–internal rotation (A–B)

Components
  Range + to +++

Notes

These activities can be performed during the early repair phase when the person is advised to minimize weight-bearing

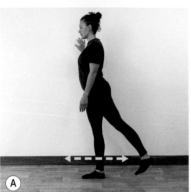

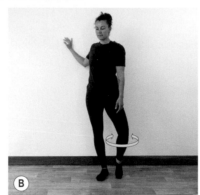

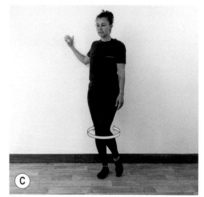

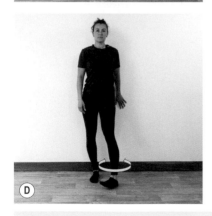

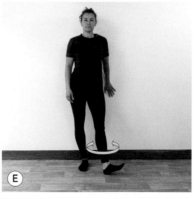

FIGURE 14.13

Description

Off-weight-bearing hip pendulum swings:
  Flexion–extension (A)
  Adduction–abduction and internal–external rotation (B–C)
  Internal–external rotation in flexion (D–E)

Components
  Range + to ++++

Notes

These activities can be performed during the early repair phase when the person is advised to minimize weight-bearing on the affected limb.

Body weight and balance can be supported by the unaffected side and by holding on to another base (crutches, holding on to a wall, chair, etc.)

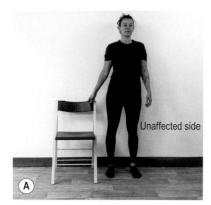
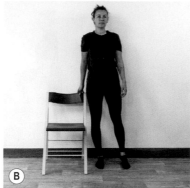
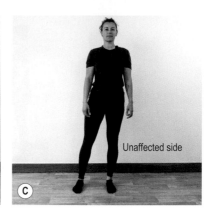
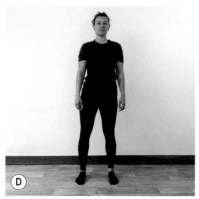
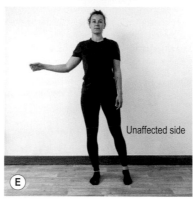

FIGURE 14.14

Description

Graded weight-bearing on the affected side, with support (A–B)

Variation: add forward and back steps with the affected limb

Weight-bearing without support, mainly on the affected side (C), equally on both sides (D), and favoring the affected side by reaching activities on the affected side (E)

Components

Loading of joints + to +++

Notes

This challenge can be used to demonstrate to the patient that weight-bearing is safe after a period of immobilization

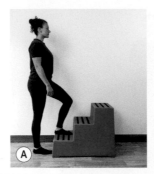 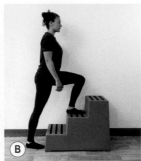

FIGURE 14.15

Description

Pre-stair-climbing lower limb movement challenges. Weight supported, with affected side raised and lower foot 1 step (A), then 2 steps (B) away; repeat this cycle several times. Use full weight-bearing on affected side as condition improves

Flexion of the knee and hip and dorsiflexion of the foot are challenged when the affected leg is leading the movement

Extension of these joints and dorsiflexion are challenged when the unaffected limb is leading the step movement. Instruct the patient to keep the heel in contact with the floor in the affected weight-bearing leg

Components

Range +++ (flexion)

Notes

Suggest this activity when the patient is passing by a staircase

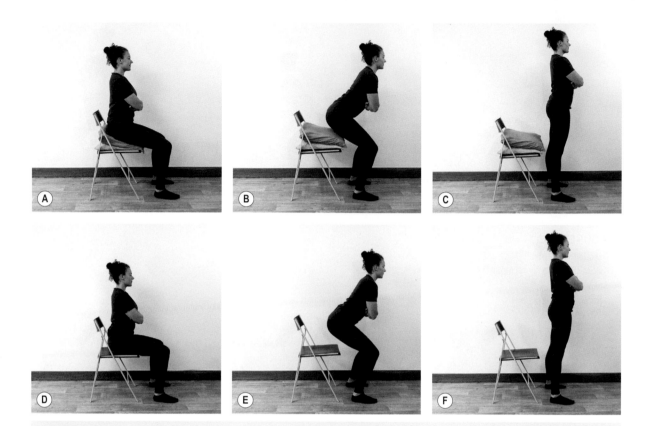

FIGURE 14.16

Description

Gradual challenge sit-to-stand from raised surface (A–C) to seat level (D–F), without support of the arms

Components

Range +++ to ++++

Force +++ to +++++

Notes

Find the height at which the patient can raise themselves without use of the arms. At home, place pillows on a couple of commonly used chairs.

Try to get 10–20 repetitions 3 times per day

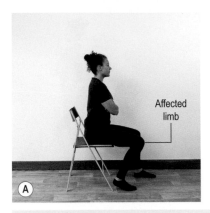
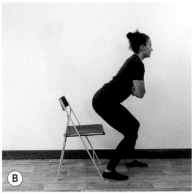
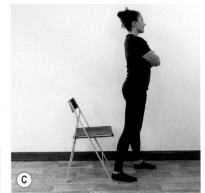

Affected limb

FIGURE 14.17

Description

Sit-to-stand from normal height but with affected knee in greater flexion

Components

Range +++ to ++++ (flexion)

Force +++ to +++++

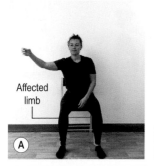
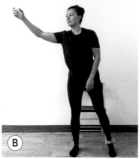

Affected limb

FIGURE 14.18

Description

Sit-to-stand from normal height while reaching sideways towards the affected side

Components

Range +++ to ++++ (flexion)

Force +++ to +++++

Notes

This provides a greater force challenge to the affected limb

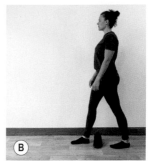

FIGURE 14.19

Description

Step repeatedly over an obstacle with affected limb (range challenge)

Step leading with unaffected limb (balance challenge)

Obstacle can be raised or placed further forward to increase the range challenge

Components

Range +++ (extension)

Force +++ to ++++ (static)

Balance/postural steadiness ++++

Notes

For safety, practice in hallway or near support

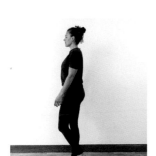
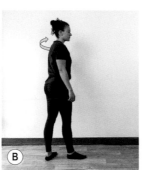

FIGURE 14.20

Description

Walk and turn

Components

Postural steadiness/balance +++++

Organization duration +++++

Range (hip rotation) +++ to +++++

Notes

Practice in hallway or walking around a table. For safety, turn towards the wall or table

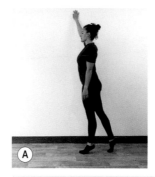
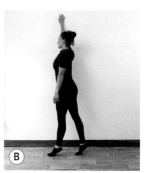

FIGURE 14.21

Description

Knee and hip extension and ankle dorsiflexion

Walking along a wall while drawing an imaginary line high above the head. Walk on forefoot

Components

Range +++++ (extension hip and knee, plantar flexion ankle/foot)

Force + to ++

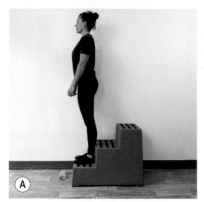
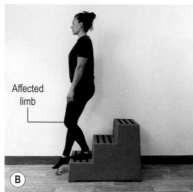
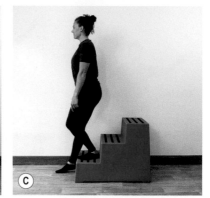

FIGURE 14.22

Description

Challenging knee and ankle ROM and force

Supported, stand on affected side. With unaffected leg, reach with the foot to an object placed on the floor (reduces the height of the step) (A–B), and back to the stair. As the patient improves, take a full step down to floor level (C); repeat several times

Components

Range + to +++ (flexion)

Range ++++ to +++++ (extension)

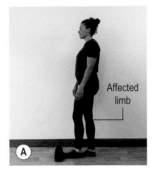
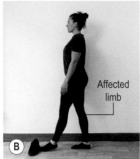
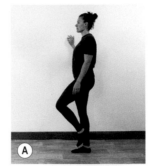
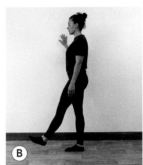

Affected limb

Affected limb

FIGURE 14.23

Description
Balance and stability using an external goal
Push obstacle along the floor with the unaffected side, while keeping the foot off the floor

Components
Range +++ (extension)
Force +++ to ++++
Balance/postural steadiness +++++
Coordination ++++++

Notes
Practice in hallway or near support

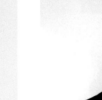

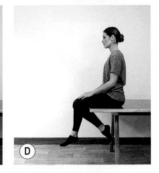

FIGURE 14.24

Description
Off-weight-bearing knee pendulum swings in standing and sitting. Flexion–extension cycles

Components
Range + to ++++

Notes
Due to swelling in the joint the patient may find 90° flexion difficult. In this situation start the pendulum swings in standing

Head and neck

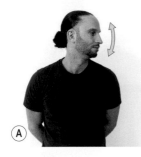

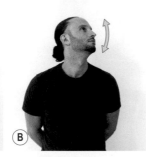

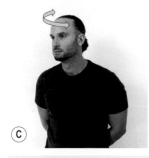

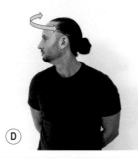

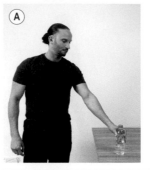

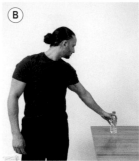

FIGURE 14.25

Description

Range desensitization for persistent stiff and painful neck.

Can be used for acute phase as movement stimulation to support repair

Rotate head to sensitive and stiff end-range, then add head movement:

Nodding flexion–extension cycles ("yes–yes" nodding) (A–B)

Nodding in rotation cycles at end-range ("no–no" nodding) (C–D)

Components

Range +++++ (rotation) with either flexion–extension or rotation cycles superimposed

Notes

Much of the recovery with chronic neck pain is associated with range desensitization

FIGURE 14.26

Description

Range desensitization using head rotation combined with a reaching-back task

Components

Range + to +++++ (rotation)

Notes

Using the arm to reach while turning the head seems to change the rotation dynamics with greater neck rotation towards the target

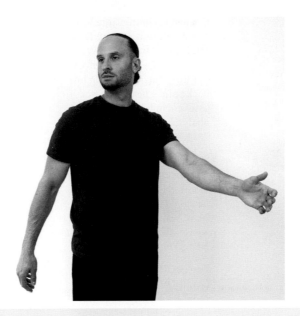

FIGURE 14.27

Description

Range desensitization

Rotate head to stiff/painful end-range and swing arm as during walking. Can be integrated into walking (this challenge brings about counter-rotation between the head and thoracic mass, resulting in rhythmic neck rotation)

Components

Range + to +++++ (rotation)

Notes

If walking, stay safe by returning the head and looking forwards every few steps

References

1. Dahm KT, Brurberg KG, Jamtvedt G, Hagen KB. Advice to rest in bed versus advice to stay active for acute low-back pain and sciatica. Cochrane Database Syst Rev. 2010 Jun 16;6:CD007612.

2. Brox JI, Sørensen R, Friis A, Nygard Ø, Indahl A, Keller A, et al. Randomized clinical trial of lumbar instrumented fusion and cognitive intervention and exercises in patients with chronic low back pain and disc degeneration. Spine. 2003;28:1913–21.

3. King JC, Kelleher WJ, Stedwill JE, Talcott G. Physical limitations are not required for chronic pain rehabilitation success. Am J Phys Med Rehab. 1994;73:331–7.

4. Brox JI. Lifting with straight legs and bent spine is not bad for your back. Scand J Pain. 2018;18:563–4.

5. Coenen P, Gouttebarge V, van der Burght AS, van Dieën JH, Frings-Dresen MHW, van der Beek AJ, et al. The effect of lifting during work on low back pain: a health impact assessment based on a meta-analysis. Occ Environ Med. 2014;71 871–7.

6. St Angelo JM, Fabiano SE. Adhesive capsulitis. In: StatPearls [Internet]. Treasure Island, FL: StatPearls; 2021 May. Available from: https://www.ncbi.nlm.nih.gov/books/NBK532955/.

7. Diercks RL, Stevens M. Gentle thawing of the frozen shoulder: a prospective study of supervised neglect versus intensive physical therapy in seventy-seven patients with frozen shoulder syndrome followed up for two years. J Shoulder Elbow Surg. 2004;13:499–502.

8. Uhthoff HK, Boileau P. Primary frozen shoulder: global capsular stiffness versus localized contracture. Clin Orthop Relat Res. 2007;456:79–84.

9. Kilian O, Kriegsmann J, Berghäuser K, Stahl JP, Horas U, Heerdegen R. The frozen shoulder: arthroscopy, histological findings and transmission electron microscopy imaging. Chirurg. 2001;72:1303–8.

10. Neer CS 2nd, Satterlee CC, Dalsey RM, Flatow EL. The anatomy and potential effects of contracture of the coracohumeral ligament. Clin Orthop Related Res. 1992;280:182–5.

11. Jain TK, Sharma NK. The effectiveness of physiotherapeutic interventions in treatment of frozen shoulder/adhesive capsulitis: a systematic review. J Back Musculoskelet Rehabil. 2014;27:247–73.

FIGURE 2.2

Forces exerted on the knee during daily and recreational activities. (Adapted from Kutzner I, Heinlein B, Graichen F, Bender A, Rohlmann A, Halder A, et al. Loading of the knee joint during activities of daily living measured in vivo in five subjects. J Biomech. 2010;43:2164–73; and D'Lima DD, Steklov N, Patil S, Colwell CW. The Mark Coventry Award: in vivo knee forces during recreation and exercise after knee arthroplasty. Clin Orthop Relat Res. 2008;466:2605–11.)

FIGURE 2.3

Forces exerted on the glenohumeral joint during daily activities. (Adapted from Bergmann G, Graichen F, Bender A, Kääb M, Rohlmann A, Westerhoff P. In vivo glenohumeral contact forces: measurements in the first patient 7 months postoperatively. J Biomech. 2007;40:2139–49.)

FIGURE 2.6

Context principle in constructing a functional exercise rehabilitation. (A) For the lower limb. (B) For the spine/trunk. (A and B, After Lederman E. Neuromuscular rehabilitation in manual and physical therapy. Edinburgh: Churchill Livingstone; 2010.)

FIGURE 4.3

Tensile strength of muscle, connective tissue, and skin after surgical repair in animals. Clinically, these time scales are highly variable and depend on numerous factors, such as the extent of damage, tissue affected, patient age, and health status. (After Kääriäinen M, Kääriäinen J, Järvinen TL, Sievänen H, Kalimo H, Järvinen M. Correlation between biomechanical and structural changes during the regeneration of skeletal muscle after laceration injury. J Orthop Res. 1998;16: 197–206; Gelberman RH, Woo SL-Y, Lothringer K, Akeson WH, Amiel D. Effects of early intermittent passive mobilization on healing canine flexor tendons. J Hand Surg. 1982;7:170–5; and Ireton JE, Unger JG, Rohrich RJ. The role of wound healing and its everyday application in plastic surgery: a practical perspective and systematic review. Plast Reconstr Surg Glob Open. 2013;1:e10–e19.)

FIGURE 4.4

Flow through the interstitium is enhanced by intermittent forces that deform the tissue. (After Benias PC, Wells RG, Sackey-Aboagye B, Klavan H, Reidy J, Buonocuore D, et al. Structure and distribution of an unrecognized interstitium in human tissues. Sci Rep. 2018;8:4947.)

FIGURE 4.5

Lymph flow is elevated by exercise intensity. (After Desai P, Williams AG Jr, Prajapati P, Downey HF. Lymph flow in instrumented dogs varies with exercise intensity. Lymphat Res Biol. 2010;8:143–8.)

FIGURE 4.6

(A) Reorganisation of the capillary bed after injury is directed by the physical forces imposed on the area by movement, demonstrated in a laboratory sample. In the unloaded model, the capillary bed is disorganized. With low load and static stretching there is progressive microvessel sprouting and organization along the force vectors in the tissue. (After Krishnan L, Underwood CJ, Maas S, Ellis BJ, Kode TC, Hoying JB, et al. Effect of mechanical boundary conditions on orientation of angiogenic microvessels. Cardiovasc Res. 2008;78:324–32.) (B) Lymphatic regeneration after injury is guided by fluid flow through the interstitium. (After Boardman KC, Swartz MA. Interstitial flow as a guide for lymphangiogenesis. Circ Res. 2003;92: 801–8.)

FIGURE 4.8

Tensile strength of repaired tendon after immobilization, delayed mobilization, and early mobilization (using passive motion). (After Gelberman RH, Woo SL-Y, Lothringer K, Akeson WH, Amiel D. Effects of early intermittent passive mobilization on healing canine flexor tendons. J Hand Surg. 1982;7:170–5.)

FIGURE 4.15

Voluntary exercise increases axonal regeneration in sensory neurons. (After Molteni R, Zheng JQ, Ying Z, Gómez-Pinilla F, Twiss JF. Voluntary exercise increases axonal regeneration from sensory neurons. Proc Natl Acad Sci U S A. 2004;101:8473-8.)

FIGURE 8.5

Recruitment specificity (electromyelogram) of anterior trunk muscles during bending. RA, rectus abdominis; EO, external oblique; IO, internal oblique; TrA, transversus abdominis. (After Carpenter MG, Tokuno CD, Thorstensson A, Cresswell AG. Differential control of abdominal muscles during multi-directional support-surface translations in man. Exper Brain Res. 2008;188:445.)

FIGURE 8.6

(A) An attempt to depict the task component profile in the legs during different activities in comparison to walking (dashed outline). (B) Different activities have their specific force-generation profiles. This can be observed to some extent in the ratio of the cross-sectional area between fast and slow muscle fibers in athletes participating in different sporting activities. Quadriceps biopsies were compared to sedentary controls. (After Goldspink G. Malleability of the motor system: a comparative approach. J Exper Biol. 1985;115:375–91.)

FIGURE 10.4

Sensitization and pain of fatigue in individuals with chronic trapezius pain. Both pain and pain-free groups experience the pain of fatigue during a light repetitive task. However, the pain group starts off with a higher level of pain, which spikes during performance of the task. (After Rosendal L, Larsson B, Kristiansen J, Peolsson M, Søgaard K, Kjær M, et al. Increase in muscle nociceptive substances and anaerobic metabolism in patients with trapezius myalgia: microdialysis in rest and during exercise. Pain. 2004;112:324–34.)

FIGURE 10.5

Pooled dose–response association between prolonged standing (in minutes) and low back symptoms and lower limb symptoms (pain or discomfort, on a 0–100 scale). (After Coenen P. Associations of prolonged standing with musculoskeletal symptoms – a systematic review of laboratory studies. Gait Posture. 2017;58:310–18.)

INDEX